The Child with Abdominal Pains

JOHN APLEY

CBE, MD, FRCP

Consultant Paediatrician, Bristol

SECOND EDITION

SECOND PRINTING

BLACKWELL SCIENTIFIC PUBLICATIONS

OXFORD LONDON EDINBURGH MELBOURNE

© 1975 Blackwell Scientific Publications
Osney Mead, Oxford OX2 0EL
8 John Street, London WC1N 2ES
9 Forrest Road, Edinburgh EH1 2QH
P.O. Box 9, North Balwyn, Victoria, Australia.

ISBN 0 632 00641 2

First published 1959
Reprinted 1964
Second edition 1975
Reprinted 1978

Distributed in the United States of America by
J.B.Lippincott Company, Philadelphia
and in Canada by
J.B.Lippincott Company of Canada Ltd., Toronto

Printed and bound in Great Britain by
Billing & Sons Ltd,
Guildford, London and Worcester

Contents

Acknowledgements

It is a pleasure to acknowledge my indebtedness to colleagues who have worked with me and helped provide some of the new material in the second edition. They include Dr Barbara Hale, for her meticulous follow-up survey; Drs Diana Haslam and Grant Tulloh and Mr John Eatoff (who first developed the infra-red pupillometer) for the pupillometry methods and apparatus, and Dr Jane Robinson who carried them further; Dr D. Burman for doing the endoscopies. The Editors of the *B.M.J.* kindly gave permission to print diagrams from a published lecture.

Preface to Second Edition

When I used the words 'little belly-achers' in the very first sentence of the preface to the first edition I could not know how they would catch on. Between doctors with similar interests in various parts of the world the term has become a password—and, indeed, almost a passport to visit and discuss this global paediatric problem. One serendipity brought back from such travels is my *International Index of Sophistication:* 'The more sophisticated the country, the the more little bellyachers will it have'.

I have held out for some time against pressure to bring out a new edition; in this I was supported by friends who preferred that the original monograph should remain unchanged. It described a series of studies aimed at clarifying a subject that was irritatingly illogical and muddled, without controls or follow-up surveys, stuffed with indigestible assumptions. Now, fortunately, paediatric gourmets have become increasingly interested and the subject is being made more digestible. At the same time it is becoming more logical, so that experience can bring not only more data but greater understanding. I find recurrent abdominal pain to be one of the most attractive and stimulating ingredients of paediatric practice; it is also one of the most rewarding, especially for the clinician who is not over-mechanised and can make a satisfactory personal relationship with children as well as parents.

The main purpose of the new edition has not been merely to add a few factual items, interesting though they are; it has been rather to re-state the basic concepts, which remain substantially unchanged from the first edition but are now reinforced by new clinical observations and experimental work.

Some minor tidying and burnishing will be allowed me; I have tried not to emulate Milton who, in the *Errata* for Paradise Lost, wrote: 'For *we* read *wee*'. Where new studies and data have been added they are kept distinct from the earlier ones. Some new clinical observations will be found and several more rarities are now included.

There are two major additions. The first is a report of a long-term follow-up survey of comprehensively treated patients, to compare with the earlier untreated ones; both I believe to have been the first such surveys in the field. The second is a report on measurements of pupillary reactions, as an indication of autonomic dysfunction. The conclusions derived from various studies have been incorporated with modern concepts of conditioning and anxiety reactions to fashion tentatively a new section on 'The Pathogenesis of Recurrent Abdominal Pain'; it may possibly also stimulate new thoughts on effective treatment.

When I set out originally to try to improve my understanding of children with abdominal pains, I found it was more realistic not to try to 'cure' their pains but to help them to adapt. Now, after an experience that covers some thousands of such children, the problems grow no less varied or challenging while the approach seems to justify itself increasingly. In the first edition of this monograph I included the dire warning 'Venter praecepta non audit' (The belly will not listen to advice). Now I believe it *will* listen; but only so long as we, the advisers, go on learning about what advice to give and how to give it. Otherwise that often quoted prediction will remain true: 'Little belly-achers grow up to be big belly-achers'—and they will 'belly-ache' about more than the abdomen.

June 1974   J.A.

Preface to First Edition

It was tempting to call this monograph 'Little Belly-Achers'. I insisted on a title which emphasizes the patient, not the symptom, and alternatives like 'Children with Recurrent Abdominal Pain' are long and unwieldy. I decided against 'Little Belly-Achers' partly because it carries a suggestion of irritation on the doctor's part. If there is any irritation with a complaint which is very common, seems to go on and on, and takes up so much time, it may be increased because of the many gaps in our knowledge. Of these the self-critical doctor is well aware when trying to make a diagnosis.

The studies brought together here are the results of attempts, often with the help of colleagues, to fill some of the gaps for myself. I confess that, as a paediatrician, I started with a bias towards organic causes (and organic cures); but the accumulating evidence gradually convinced me that in most cases an organic cause cannot be found. Moreover, an organic cause cannot explain the other disturbances which are commonly associated with recurrent abdominal pain.

The reader will notice that the studies described are interspersed with controls. They were part of the process by which I tried to assess the significance of variations from the normal, and the validity of diagnoses which are currently accepted. In the haul from these turbid waters I found many red herrings.

The book is in two parts. The first, containing the bulk of the original work, includes observations on: frequency; age and sex incidence; a long-term follow-up survey; the important family history; the diagnostic value of pain and associated phenomena; an appraisal of organic disorders, with indications for ancillary investigations; a review of intellectual and emotional factors; and an assessment of treatment by drugs (including a therapeutic trial) and by other methods. I am told that readers will be well advised to read the chapter summaries first. The second part of the book is largely discussion, though a few items of original work are incorporated where they fall naturally in place. It ends with a chapter on diagnosis and management which is, in effect, a summing up.

A friendly critic likened some of the case histories to the dazzling illustrations on seed packets, as compared with the humdrum specimens we usually see. They are not touched up or toned down, but are truly representative of what is found in children with recurrent abdominal pain.

Bristol, February 1959   JOHN APLEY

Part I
Original Inquiries

Chapter 1
Problems of Recurrent Abdominal Pain in Childhood

Clinical problems. Diagnostic difficulties

It is a common event for the family doctor or paediatrician to be called to a child who complains, not for the first time, of abdominal pain. He may have been sent home from school 'because his tummy ached' and the teacher thought he looked unwell. Probably he felt sick, and he may have vomited. Usually, by the time the doctor arrives the pain has gone; but, whether the child is fully recovered or not, the parents ask questions to which answers are difficult. Even if the pain persists, the doctor may still be in the awkward position of finding nothing definite on which to base a diagnosis. Asked where the pain is, the child vaguely puts his hand on the umbilicus. Asked what it feels like, he replies simply 'It hurts'. He may look pale, the tongue is usually clean, the pulse unaffected, and the temperature normal or somewhat raised. All that is to be discovered on examination is, as a rule, indefinite tenderness in the abdomen.

If he knows the family well the doctor may appreciate that this is not an isolated disturbance. Not only has the child had pain before but, as likely as not, the mother or father has a history of a similar complaint—there may even be an abdominal scar to show for it. He may realize that the child, and indeed the family, tends to be over-controlled or 'to get worked up'. Usually, and shrewdly, he decides that he can afford to await developments—but he must often feel doubts. Was his reassurance completely justified? Is he overlooking an early acute appendicitis?—should he have carried out further investigations or sent the child to hospital?—was sedation the best form of treatment? And if there is, as he expects, a quick recovery, what of the future?

These interrelated problems—of aetiology, clinical diagnosis, indications for investigation, methods of treatment, and prognosis

3

—are even commoner than is generally realized: at least one school child in ten suffers from recurrent abdominal pain (p. 23). Moreover, as the discussion on prognosis and natural history indicates (p. 17), the disorder is far from being so self-limited (or benign) as is still often accepted.

DIAGNOSTIC DIFFICULTIES

Diagnosis passes through phases which reflect changing medical fashions. In 'Common Disorders and Diseases of Children' Still (1909) wrote: 'I know of no symptom which can be more obscure in its causation than colicky abdominal pain in childhood', and listed various causes. The commonest he thought to be some form of 'indigestion', then followed: undigested vegetable matter, threadworms, simple constipation, nervous bowel, renal disorders, tuberculous adhesions or caseating glands and appendicitis. In the second edition (1912) of his book he added 'abdominal epilepsy', also on evidence which by modern standards is open to criticism. Some of these possibilities have been discarded, others retained or revived, while new ones are added from time to time. Among the hardy perennials are worms, chronic or 'grumbling' appendicitis and mesenteric adenitis. Among more recent crops of diagnoses are allergy, emotional disorders, virus infections, hypoglycaemia, the periodic syndrome and abdominal migraine; others, like dietary or dental faults and acidosis, are at present out of favour.

Like other medical problems, that of recurrent abdominal pain has many facets, and in a large number of investigations attention has been focused on one to the virtual exclusion of the remainder. Even in the small number of more comprehensive inquiries, however, there is often apparent a tendency to selection of cases and, a very conspicuous omission, an absence of 'controls'.

Accurate criteria on which to base diagnosis have not been clearly established. In consequence doctors tend to vacillate between two extremes: simply to dismiss recurrent abdominal pains as an insoluble problem or, alternatively, to indulge in diagnostic aids without adequate justification. It is interesting and instructive to speculate on possible reasons for the diagnostic difficulties.

By training, and perhaps by inclination, most clinicians seize on an abnormal physical sign almost with a feeling of relief. An abnormality which can be seen, felt, or heard affords the same sort of satisfaction as playing games: the pitch is marked out and the rules are known; the linesmen are our technical colleagues (laboratory and X-ray) and the referee is the morbid pathologist. From this attitude certain consequences derive.

History-taking. The form of history-taking which clinicians customarily adopt in practice is biased towards eliciting evidence of organic disease. But in dealing with children suffering from recurrent abdominal pain its shortcomings are repeatedly made evident. In the large majority of cases a history limited in this way proves unproductive, and a considerable broadening of the approach is clearly essential if a reliable diagnosis is to be made on evidence that is logical and consistent.

Physical examination. In practice, the attempt to make a diagnosis often leads, not unnaturally, to repeated and more thorough physcial examinations. But extremely few children with recurrent abdominal pain have a clinically detectable physical abnormality (Chap. 5).

Even if one is found, however, diagnosis can become more, not less, difficult; for some of the abnormalities may mistakenly be considered to explain the pains, though in fact they do not. I refer to such conditions as grossly defective teeth or poor posture, which may be termed 'false positives'. They may be corrected or neglected: the pains may cease or persist. Too often an abnormality is accepted as causative without proof.

Ancillary investigations. Sometimes, especially in children attending hospital, the next stage is to set out on a witch-hunt of ancillary investigations. Appetite may grow with what it feeds on. If one test is negative more and more may be invoked. Even if a test is admittedly inconclusive it is sometimes accepted *faute de mieux* and a complete structure of disorder erected on this foundation. Furthermore, some of the abnormalities revealed by ancillary investigations are on a par with the 'false positives' of physical examination. Thus, the detection of worms in the stools, radiological evidence of calcified tuberculous lymph nodes in the abdomen, or reports of abnormal electroencephalographic tracings, may be actively misleading. They should not be accepted as indicating a cause for the symptom without knowing what is found in symptom-free children, and the whole context of what might be elicited from the individual child.

Results of treatment. Finally, the apparent success of a particular form of treatment, i.e. the cessation of pain, must not be un-critically accepted as proof either of the diagnosis or the theory of causation. The history of this complaint follows a recognized pattern in that a succession of different remedies has seemed for a time to produce 'cures'; in retrospect their apparent, if possibly transient, effectiveness appears to depend largely on the doctor's conviction that he is right.

Chapter 2
Materials and Methods
of Inquiry

Criteria. Hospital Series, School Series and School Control Series.
Additional material. History, examination and ancillary
investigations

The type of case to be included under the term 'recurrent abdominal pain' was defined, and the criteria were applied to the main groups of children studied in hospital or at school.

Criteria
Those included were children who had complained of at least three episodes of pain, severe enough to affect their activities, over a period longer than three months. Those excluded (a very small proportion of the number seen) were: children under the age of 3 years, those in whom pain had not recurred during the year prior to being questioned, and those who came unattended by a parent.

These criteria were defined, first, to ensure a reasonable degree of accuracy in the history; and, second, to eliminate, on the one hand, trivial disturbances (such as isolated digestive upsets) or, on the other, serious diseases (including occult infection) which would be expected to become manifest within the time limits set. In the event, the limitations imposed rarely raised any difficulties as regards selection of cases.

Data were obtained from two main groups of children (additional material is indicated on p. 11).

Hospital Series
The first group will be referred to as the Hospital Series.

A comprehensive study was made of a hundred consecutive children referred to hospital with recurrent abdominal pain as the main symptom.

7

There are, however, two obvious disadvantages of such a method by itself: children referred to hospital form a selected and not necessarily representative group, and a valid comparison with healthy controls is not feasible.

School Series and Controls

For these reasons, in a second group (termed the School Series) a limited study of unselected school children was undertaken. This also provided material for assessing the incidence of the complaint.

Under the aegis of a City Local Authority, children from Primary and Secondary Modern Schools regularly attend with a parent for routine Medical Examinations. For a period of more than a year, at some of these clinics chosen at random, all children attending (and their parents) were questioned regarding the occurrence of abdominal pain. Each child in whom the criteria set out above were satisfied was included in the School Series.

The child not complaining of abdominal pain, whose name happened to be next on the list of those attending, was examined and included in the Control Series. The number of controls was however, augmented by adding further children at random, as often as time permitted, and by including a small number below school age who by chance had come with their parents.

The investigation was concluded when 1000 children with their parents had been questioned, and has been reported in full elsewhere (Apley and Naish, 1958). The material is summarized in Table 1.

Table 1. School series and controls: case material

	Total	Boys	Girls
Preliminary questioning	1000	528	472
Detailed questioning and examination:			
Children with recurrent abdominal pain*	108	50	58
Controls	312	155	157

* Thirteen children whose pains had ceased more than a year previously have been excluded here and from the calculations of incidence.

CHILDREN WITH PAIN

In both the Hospital Series and the School Series the history was taken and the clinical examination carried out on identical lines.

Family history. In eliciting the family history special attention was paid to the occurrence of abdominal pain in other members of the family, as well as to migraine, epilepsy, allergic, 'nervous' and other disorders.

Personal history. The personal history was obtained from the mother as well as from the child. An accurate description of pain in children may be difficult or impossible to obtain, but detailed inquiries were made regarding several aspects in particular. They included the time and mode of onset of the attacks of pain, and any changes occurring subsequently; their site, character, duration, time of occurrence and periodicity; and any predisposing and alleviating factors. Associated phenomena like vomiting, headache, pyrexia and pallor, and sleepiness after attacks were noted. An attempt was made to gauge the severity of the pain, and its effect on the child's activities, as well as the child's reaction to pain in general. Questions were asked about diet and appetite; dizziness, blank turns, faint spells, fits and other obvious indications of epilepsy; psychological disturbances, and evidence of emotional tension, both at home and at school.

Examination. The physical examination was detailed and as complete as possible. A number of children in the Hospital Series were again examined during an attack of pain, when particular attention was paid to the child's general appearance, the site of the pain, the size of the abdomen, the abdominal wall, the presence of bowel sounds and the plantar reflexes. The psychological status and the intellectual status were estimated, and the assessment checked where possible by reports from the school authorities.

Ancillary investigations. It is generally agreed that over-investigation may prove harmful. Nevertheless, organic disease should be promptly excluded or confirmed, and for this purpose 'screening' investigations may be necessary. One of the objects of the present study was to try to determine the indications for specific investigations. A large proportion of those carried out was found to be unnecessary, and would not be advocated in everyday practice. What William Penn termed 'a wantonness in inquiry' must be avoided. The very small number which were found to be essential are indicated on p. 104.

The ancillary investigations carried out in the original Hospital Series are summarized in Table 6. Routine procedures were: Mantoux test (1/1000), urinalysis (macroscopic and microscopic), blood count, electroencephalogram (E.E.G.), and plain radiograph of the abdomen. Some additional investigations were carried out as 'pilot' surveys. Thus, in a proportion of cases the following were done: stool examination and rectal smear (for ova, worms and eosinophils), urine examination (for porphyrins), liver function tests, skin and serological tests (for brucellosis), pyelography, radiology of the intestine with complete barium follow-through examination (both between and during attacks of pain). With the weight of accumulating evidence some of these were abandoned as routine even for the purpose of the survey, and were subsequently employed only for specific indications.*

In theory it might have seemed more satisfactory to carry out similar investigations on children in the School Series. In practice, however, this was considered to be not only impracticable but also undesirable. The only ancillary investigation carried out in the School Series was electroencephalography (E.E.G.).

Controls
The method of selection of controls in the School Series has been outlined (p. 8). In those selected a detailed history was obtained and clinical examination carried out in the same way as for the children with pain. In a high proportion of these controls an E.E.G. was obtained, but no further investigations were carried out.

In the Hospital Series the results of some examinations and investigations (e.g. plain radiograph of the abdomen, E.E.G., intelligence assessment, etc.) were compared with those obtained from children attending hospital for some reason other than abdominal pain. They will be discussed under the appropriate headings. A therapeutic trial will also be described.

---

* Subsequently pilot surveys, each of up to 20 cases, have been undertaken or lactose intolerance and for antibodies to brucella and to toxocara infections. All were non-productive. In a small number of additional cases endoscopy (page 98) has been carried out.

COMPARISON BETWEEN SCHOOL SERIES AND HOSPITAL SERIES

The children forming both the School Series and Hospital Series were drawn from working and middle-class families in a large city, with a population approaching half a million and negligible unemployment. The Hospital Series included in addition a small proportion of patients from the surrounding country districts. From the inquiries made, milk-drinking habits appeared to be similar in the two groups, and the investigations done precluded the possibility that predominantly rural diseases (e.g. brucellosis) might have weighted the Hospital Series unduly.

A comparison of the data from the School Series and the Hospital Series showed only a few minor differences, the significance of which will be discussed later. In brief, the Hospital Series included proportionately more children in whom attacks of pain were severe, more 'only children', rather more with epileptiform E.E.G.s, and fewer girls in the pre-pubertal age-group. Under the major headings of family and personal history, and physical, mental and psychological status, the data from the two groups showed a close similarity, and the material forming the two Series did not differ in any important respect.

Additional material
Some addition smaller groups of cases were investigated for special purposes. They are described in the text, where they fall naturally in the sequence of investigations and discussion. Examples are: (1) long-term follow-up survey (p. 18), (2) calcification of mesenteric nodes (p. 37), (3) E.E.G. in children with pain and in controls (p. 39), (4) virus studies (p. 78), (5) pains in epileptic children (p. 87).

In addition, as a measure of autonomic function, pupillometry has now been done on a group of children and some parents (page 99). In a further group the pain threshold was estimated (page 26).

Summary
Criteria for inclusion of cases. In children 3 years of age or more:
(1) At least three attacks of pain. (2) Pain severe enough to affect

activities. (3) Attacks recurring over a period longer than 3 months, and continuing in the year prior to the investigation.

Material of the inquiry. In two main groups of children, at hospital and school respectively, the history was obtained and physical examination carried out according to the same schedule.

(a) *Hospital Series.* In a hundred consecutive children ancillary investigations were carried out. Wherever possible, the findings were compared with those from children not complaining of abdominal pain.

(b) *School Series and School Controls.* A thousand unselected school-children (and their parents) were questioned. In those with recurrent abdominal pain satisfying the above criteria the history and clinical findings were recorded. A large number of randomly selected children, similarly questioned and examined, formed a control series. In a large proportion of those with or without pain E.E.G.s were obtained.

The data of history and clinical examination from the Hospital and the School Series were compared in detail and showed close similarity.

(c) *Additional material.* Several additional groups of children were studied for special purposes.

Chapter 3
The Family and the Child:
Medical History, Prognosis and
Natural History

*Familial incidence of recurrent abdominal pain and
of other disorders. Previous illness in the child. Prognosis
and Natural History: long-term inquiry*

The family doctor, it has been neatly said: 'Is a naturalist, pursuing his quarry and studying its habits in the jungle: the specialist only the specimens in the zoo.' The proper study for every doctor is not merely a symptom, organ, region or disease, but the whole patient, in the background of the family and the environment. Pain is an experience in which the whole patient takes part.

This chapter presents data from the medical histories of the families and of the children who complained of abdominal pain.

THE FAMILY

When tuberculosis or another infection is discovered in a child it is necessary to inquire about the health of the family: it is no less important to do so with recurrent abdominal pain.

Detailed inquiries were made regarding the occurrence of abdominal pain and other complaints in the families of children with pain (School Series) and the results compared with those of similar inquiries in the families of controls (School Controls). As a further check, the families of children with pain from both the School Series and the Hospital Series were compared: it was found that in these two groups the data were closely similar.

Familial incidence of recurrent abdominal pain
In the parents and siblings of children with recurrent abdominal

pain, the incidence of similar complaints was nearly six times higher than in those of controls (Table 2). The member of the family most often affected was the mother. In several families two or three members were affected.

Details regarding relatives (cousins, grandparents, uncles and aunts) outside the immediate family were harder to come by, and were not considered sufficiently exact to warrant statistical presentation. Nevertheless, the incidence was several times higher in the relatives of children with abdominal pain than in the relatives of controls.

Familial incidence of other disorders
The incidence of other common disorders in the families of children with recurrent abdominal pain was compared with the incidence in controls (Table 3).

Included under 'peptic ulcer' were only those who were said to have had radiological confirmation, a haematemesis or operation;

Table 2. History of recurrent abdominal pain in the families of schoolchildren

| | Percentage affected in families | |
Relation	of children without pain	of children with pain
Sibling	4	18
Mother	2	17
Father	2	11
Total	8	46

under 'migraine' all severe headaches*; and under 'nervous breakdown' disorders severe enough to have caused a serious disruption of normal life. The information on which these diagnoses were listed was obtained from non-medical sources, and cannot be claimed as exact, though this qualification applies equally to both groups. The figures for 'fits' are too small to be statistically evaluable, but the families of children with pain showed a significant preponderance of the other disorders listed.

* But see p. 102 for the results from further questioning.

For further disorders, including tuberculosis, the allergic group, psychoses, and serious behaviour disturbances, the numbers were extremely small and no obvious differences between the two groups emerged.

Table 3. Other disorders in the families of schoolchildren

History of:	Percentage affected in families of children without pain	of children with pain
Peptic ulcer	3	10*
Appendicectomy	3	8
Migraine	3	14
Nervous breakdown	2	10
Fits	3	6

* Two parents had suffered from recurrent abdominal pain since childhood.

Other familial factors
In the type of inquiry undertaken it was not possible to investigate such factors as economic and housing conditions. An attempt was made to ascertain the number of 'broken homes' (with one or both parents dead, or permanently or frequently away from home) in the families of children with and without pain respectively, but the figures were too small for justifiable conclusions.

The very important aspect of emotional disturbances in the family is considered later (Chap. 6).

Position in the family
There was no apparent association between the child's numerical position in the family and a liability to abdominal pain. The proportion of 'only children' with pain was 14 per cent in the School Series, and 22 per cent in the Hospital Series, as against 12 per cent in the School Controls. From this it may be inferred that an only child with recurrent abdominal pain is more likely to be referred to hospital with this complaint than is one of several children in a family.

THE CHILD

Past history

Details of the past history were compared in children with and without recurrent abdominal pain, and some important data are shown in Table 4.

Table 4. Past history of illness in schoolchildren

	Percentage in children	
	without pain	with pain
Tonsillectomy	26	24
Appendicectomy	0.3	5
Frequent headaches	5	14
Bilious attacks	5	12
Habitual constipation	3	5
Fits	6	2
Asthma	2	6

No significant differences were elicited as regards the incidence of serious illnesses in general, head injuries, or predisposition to upper respiratory infections. The tonsillectomy rate was almost the same in the two groups.

The comparatively high appendicectomy rate in children with recurrent abdominal pain is of interest. The relevant histories of all five children with a history of appendicectomy were obtained and are summarized herewith.

Case 1. Colicky pains for 9 months. 'Normal-looking appendix' removed. Pains recurred.

Case 2. Pains for several months. Operation performed because of tenderness in R. iliac fossa. Normal appendix removed. Pains recurred.

Case 3. Pains for several years. 'Mildly infected appendix' removed. No further pains when seen 2 years later.

Case 4. No previous pains. Operation at 2 years of age: pelvic abscess and acutely inflamed appendix which was removed. Recurrent abdominal pains in the ensuing 7 years.

Case 5. Four attacks of abdominal pain in 2 years. In the fifth attack pain became localized for the first time in the R. iliac fossa, with overlying rigidity. Acutely inflamed retro-caecal appendix removed. No further history available.

In the Hospital Series, too, appendicectomy had been performed in 5 per cent of cases.

In four the appendix was not inflamed. In the fifth an acutely inflamed appendix had been removed in the first attack of abdominal pain; when seen 3 years later the child had continued to suffer from recurrent abdominal pain. Clinical examination and ancillary investigations were then negative, but there was positive evidence of considerable emotional disturbance and over-dependence on the mother.

Children with recurrent abdominal pain were significantly more liable than were the controls to frequent headaches and to bilious attacks (cyclical vomiting).

For constipation, and for asthma (and other disorders with a possible allergic basis), there was a slight preponderance in the group of children with pain, but the numbers are too small to be significant. Among children with pain, there were fewer with a history of fits than among the controls; but again the numbers are small, and the incidence of 'fainting', blank or dizzy spells and the like did not differ in the two groups.

Prognosis and Natural History

An impression that children with recurrent abdominal pain will 'grow out of it' is widely held. I have been unable to find any recorded facts either to confirm or refute it.*

* Follow-up reports which have since come to my notice are summarized. *Heinild et al. (1959)—Denmark.* A predominantly radiological report. 135 children had x-ray examination of the stomach and duodenum and 81 were re-examined after 3 years. Commonly occurring mucosal changes and increased peristalsis are described; these often persisted even though the pains were improved or gone. One of the original 135 patients had an ulcer crater and this persisted at follow-up.

Friedman (1972)—U.S.A. A report based on mailed questionnaires which were posted 1 to 3 years after initial examination of 74 children. There were 64 replies. Among these 69 per cent were reported to be free of pains or much improved, 22 per cent slightly improved, 9 per cent not improved or worse.

Keynan et al. (1973)—Israel. 40 children who had been hospitalized for abdominal pain were interviewed at least 5 years later. Five were reported to show organic disease (3 peptic ulcer, 1 familial Mediterranean fever, 1 pyloric stenosis). 12 still complained of abdominal pain and 'several others of various symptoms'.

Papatheophilou et al. (1972)—England. Predominantly an EEG survey (see pages 40 and 90).

Retrospectively, it is recognized that some adults with peptic ulcer give a history of abdominal pains since childhood (two such cases are included in Table 3); that migraine in adults is sometimes preceded by recurrent vomiting or abdominal pain, or both, in childhood; and that the 'inadequacy' of adults (who react to stress by complaining of bodily symptoms) may be established in the early years of life. But the validity of these observations, as applied to children with abdominal pain, has not been assessed; and information on which to base prognosis and a Natural History is lacking. A major difficulty is to observe, from childhood into adult life, a considerable number of cases which are both unselected and untreated. Though limited in scope, the inquiry (Apley and Naish, 1959) summarized below does, however, show trends so definite that conclusions may justifiably be drawn.

Long-term inquiry

Information was obtained, in the first instance, about the progress of eighteen patients who, as children, had attended a hospital with the complaint of recurrent abdominal pain. Attacks of pain had occurred over a period of at least 3 months before they were examined and investigated. In none had an organic cause for the symptom been found. A few had been treated with preparations of belladonna, rhubarb and the like for a short period, but most were untreated. All ceased attending hospital very soon after the possibility of organic disease was discounted.

Between 9 and 20 years later a colleague or I visited their homes to make inquiries, and further necessary details were obtained from the family doctors and hospitals.

Similar inquiries were made about eighteen 'controls'. These were randomly selected cases, matched with the previous group as closely as possible for age and sex, who had attended the same hospital at about the same period with trivial disorders.

CASES WITH RECURRENT ABDOMINAL PAIN IN
CHILDHOOD

Bodily symptoms. The findings are summarized in Table 5.

In ten of the eighteen cases abdominal pains had ceased (Group I). In two they ceased immediately after attending hospital, and in the remainder after periods varying from 2 to 12 years. In four cases, however, other recurrent symptoms had developed, among which headache (possibly migrainous in two) was the commonest.

In eight of the eighteen cases attacks of recurrent abdominal pain persisted (Group II), though usually they had become less frequent and less severe. (It is important to note that in two cases pains ceased for a few years, but recurred at 17 or 18 years of age.) Four of the eight cases now complained also of recurrent headache, and two of typical migraine (occurring independently of attacks of abdominal pain).

Nervous disorders. The incidence of nervous disorders was high, though a marked difference was found between the two groups.

Among the ten cases in whom abdominal pains had ceased, the majority (seven cases) seemed satisfactorily adjusted from the psychological point of view.

Among the eight cases in whom pains continued, only two seemed reasonably well adjusted. The remaining six had nervous and emotional disturbances of varying degrees of severity.

CONTROLS

Among the controls, one complained of moderate or severe headaches (and four of slight occasional headaches), three of occasional abdominal discomfort (associated with over-eating in one, eating ice-cream in one and constipation in the third), and one from a broken home had suffered from 'bad nerves' all her life.

ADDITIONAL CASES

In a further twelve cases, who in childhood had attended hospital with recurrent abdominal pain, inquiries similar to the above were made through the family doctor. Information in the patients' records was amplified as the result of a visit by the doctor to the patient's home for the purpose. The inquiries were carried out between 8 and 12 years after the hospital attendance, the ages of the patients then ranging between 15 and 23 years.

Three patients were completely symptom-free (pains in one case had ceased after appendicectomy).

In five cases attacks of abdominal pain had ceased, but they had other complaints: typical migraine in one, severe headaches in two, headaches with other symptoms in two. Two had some form of 'nerves'.

In four cases recurrent abdominal pain persisted (having recurred in two cases after an interval of a few years). All complained,

Table 5. Children with recurrent abdominal pain. Long-term inquiry

	Age at onset	Age at inquiry	At age	Group I Abdominal pains ceased Subsequent symptoms	Group II Abdominal pains continuing Changes in symptoms
Boys					
1	3	15	13	Frequent headache, sometimes followed by vomiting	
2	4	17	4	NONE*	
3	4	24	16	NONE	
4	6	19			Occasional vertigo. Pains usually milder, but last attack very severe
5	6	15	8	Leg and thigh pains	
6	7	20	11	NONE	
7	9	21			Perforated duodenal ulcer at 16. Monthly pains with headache
8	9	23	15	NONE	
9	9	23			Pains fewer, three or four annually. Vomiting ceased
Girls					
1	1	12			Pains less frequent and severe. Migraine attacks for 1 year
2	4	15	12	NONE	
3	4	17	11	Dysmenorrhoea, bilious attacks, headaches	
4	4	18	16	Headaches in past year	
5	4	19			Pains fewer, three or four annually. Migraine attacks past 2 years
6	7	20			Only two pains in many years. Dysmenorrhoea, nervous diarrhoea, headaches

Table 5 continued

| | | | Group I | Group II |
| | | | Abdominal pains ceased | Abdominal pains continuing |
Age at onset	Age at inquiry	At age	Subsequent symptoms	Changes in symptoms
7	7	19		Pains less severe. Vomiting ceased. Fainting, headaches
8	8	19	8 NONE	
9	8	20		Pains 'changed', less severe and frequent. Dysmenorrhoea, frequent headache

* 'NONE' does not exclude occasional mild headaches, which occurred in several cases.

in addition, of recurrent headaches, and two of severe dysmenorrhoea. One was 'neurotic' and another was 'a bad case of nerves'.

COMMENT

The natural history of recurrent abdominal pain commencing in childhood can be outlined from the thirty cases described.

In nine cases the patient became symptom-free; in nine cases attacks of abdominal pain ceased, but other symptoms developed; in twelve cases attacks of abdominal pain persisted, almost invariably with additional symptoms.

Among the twenty-one patients with continuing symptoms, three suffered from typical migraine and fifteen from moderate or severe headaches (often with other symptoms). Nervous disorders of varying severity occurred in thirteen.

These data derived from cases referred to hospital for a second opinion: the results cannot be held to apply equally to cases not so referred (possibly because the symptoms are less severe or persistent or because the family accepts them). It is, however, clear that in many cases the recurrent abdominal pains of childhood are not self-limited or, indeed, benign. Why has the not infrequent persistence, or substitution, of bodily or nervous symptoms between childhood and adult life escaped general attention? Two likely explanations may be put forward. First, because the symptoms sometimes clear up for a few years, in the adolescent period, perhaps to recur later; and second, because of the artificial separation between paediatrics and adult medicine.

From the data summarized, the long-term prognosis in children with abdominal pain appears gloomy; but the cases discussed were either untreated or inadequately treated. With rational treatment the prognosis must surely be susceptible of improvement (see pp. 58 and 105 and under Pathogenesis, p. 83).

Summary

A high incidence of abdominal pain was found in the relatives of children with recurrent abdominal pain. There was also a significantly raised incidence of peptic ulcer, headache and 'nervous breakdown', in comparison with the families of controls.

Children with recurrent abdominal pain showed an increased liability to headaches and to bilious attacks, and the appendicectomy rate was unnecessarily high.

A high proportion of adolescents and young adults, who had attended hospital with recurrent abdominal pain in childhood, were found to have continuing symptoms. Nearly half had nervous disorders. In approximately one-third of the total, attacks of abdominal pain continued (nearly always with other symptoms). In one-third abdominal pains had ceased, but other symptoms developed (the commonest was recurrent headache, and a proportion had typical migraine). Only one-third of the total number were symptom-free. In other words 'Little bellyachers are likely to grow up to be big bellyachers.'

Chapter 4
Pain and Associated Phenomena

Incidence of recurrent abdominal pain. Age at onset.
Characteristics and diagnostic significance of pain.
Associated phenomena

Incidence of recurrent abdominal pain

The incidence of recurrent abdominal pain in childhood was calculated from the investigation of 1000 unselected schoolchildren (p. 8). The over-all incidence was 10.8 per cent, with girls (12.3 per cent) more commonly affected than boys (9.5 per cent).

A still higher incidence of 'periodic abdominal pain' has since been reported (Pringle *et al.*, 1966) in this country, with 15.7 per cent of girls and 14 per cent of boys affected. These figures are taken from the invaluable National Child Development Study (1958 Cohort) in which the progress of several thousand children is being followed. The information is obtained by questionnaires and through local authorities, whereas my own data were obtained directly from parents and patients and my criteria were interpreted by one person.

Fig. 1 illustrates the variations in incidence according to age. In boys from 5 to 10 years of age there was a fairly constant incidence of between 10 per cent and 12 per cent, then a fall, followed by a late peak at 14 years. In girls the incidence was similar up to 8 years of age; but then a marked rise occurred, with more than a quarter of all girls aged 9 years affected, and subsequently a steady decrease.

The sex and age incidence in the Hospital Series followed a similar pattern, but with one difference: there were fewer girls between the ages of 8 and 10. It was inferred that they are not referred to hospitals because, at this period of their development, the symptom is accepted as trivial.

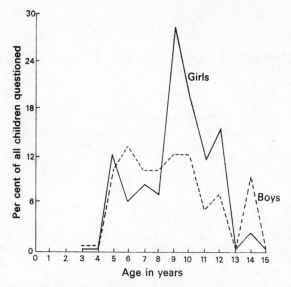

Figure 1. Proportion of schoolchildren affected at each year of age.

Age at onset of recurrent abdominal pain

The age at onset of recurrent abdominal pain in 118* children is shown diagrammatically in Fig. 2, which illustrates an interesting difference between boys and girls.

In both sexes there was a steady rise in the number of cases commencing in each year up to the age of 5. In boys the numbers then fell; but in girls there was a further striking increase, with attacks commencing in a large proportion (nearly half the total) between 8 and 10 years of age, and none subsequently.

CHARACTERISTICS OF THE PAIN

Many adults find it difficult to describe pain, and in children the difficulty is even greater. But, with patience on the doctor's part, the child can be induced to point out its site and sometimes to give

---

* This total was made up of 108 children with continuing attacks of abdominal pain, together with thirteen in whom the attacks had ceased more than a year previously, less three in whom the age at onset was not known.

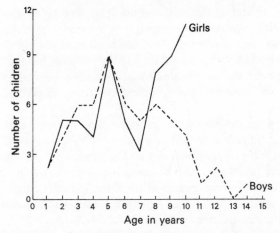

Figure 2. Age at onset of pains (118 children: 57 boys, 61 girls).

a description, at least in terms of analogy. The information is likely to be more consistent and accurate if it is obtained during, rather than between, attacks. As one little boy said, on being asked where his pain was felt: 'When I get it again I'll show you'.

The following description is based on the data obtained from children in the Hospital Series (those from the School Series corresponded quite closely).

Site. In two-thirds of the cases the pain was referred only to the region of the umbilicus. In a further 12 per cent it passed from the umbilicus to one or other side (usually the right). In another 12 per cent both umbilicus and epigastrium were indicated, and in a small number it was felt in the epigastrium alone. In the few remaining it could not be located.

The significance of location will be discussed later (p. 69), but briefly it may be stated that the common type of central abdominal pain is less likely than peripheral abdominal pain to indicate an organic disorder.

Description. In about one-third of cases the pain was described as a dull ache. In less than a third it was colicky. In the remainder it might be 'sharp as needles' or knives, gnawing, pinching, kicking, 'like a lump of food', 'like wanting to be excused', or was not described. One boy remarked 'It feels brown' and another "It feels as if someone is burning toast in my tummy'.

The character of the pain had no diagnostic significance.

Severity. An attempt was made to estimate the child's sensitiveness to pain in general. In a few with more severe abdominal pain it seemed to be increased for all forms of pain, but the difficulty of assessment was complicated by an apparent relationship between severe pain in the child and marked emotional disturbance in the mother.

Using a spring-loaded device to measure pressure exerted over the tibia, the *pain threshold* was estimated in a group of children with recurrent abdominal pain and a group without. No differences were found between the two groups. (To provide a baseline, pain thresholds were measured in normal children from 5 to 18 years (Haslam, 1969). The figures obtained showed clearly that the pain threshold rises with age.)

In nearly half the hospital cases the pain was mild, in about a quarter moderately severe, and in a quarter very severe (severe cases were, understandably, rather fewer in the School Series). The degree of severity was judged both by the description given and by the effects, e.g. whether the child stopped playing, sat or lay down, went to bed, or cried. One child in ten cried with the pain; two children (neither with a demonstrable organic disorder) screamed aloud with pain.

Many of the most severe pains were not associated with any demonstrable physical abnormality. In the very occasional case, seen over a period of many years, of a child who shrieks and writhes in pain, no organic cause has been found and I regard this as a form of hysteria. (See p. 74, under Pseudo-colic.) In the cases with organic disorders pain tended to be persistently of the same degree of severity, or of increasing severity over a long period of time. In some children without any demonstrable organic disorder there was a tendency for marked fluctuations in the severity of the pains.

Time of occurrence. In half the cases pain occurred variably at any time of day or night. In fifteen children it occurred predominantly in the mornings (in a few before breakfast); in the same number it predominated in the evening or at night. Eight children were wakened from sleep by pain. In a few an inconstant relationship with meals was described. Excitement, or worry, or 'being worked up', or vague indisposition, frequently preceded the onset of pains. In a small number of children who were in hospital, pain occurred during, or soon after, a visit from the parents.

In a high proportion of children who were wakened by pain, barium meal X-ray examination was carried out, and in many with early morning pain blood sugar estimations were obtained. In both groups the results were invariably negative.

The time of occurrence of pain could not be related to underlying organic disease.

Duration. Great variability was noted as regards the duration of pain, both from case to case and from time to time in most children considered individually. The commonest story was of frequent attacks of pain lasting for a few moments, with intervals of some minutes, the whole episode lasting for a few or many minutes. Occasionally it lasted for several hours, and rarely for several days.* A few children with mild, vague aches claimed that pain was present more often than it was absent; but their activities usually seemed unrestricted, and their appearance unaffected, even when the pain was present.

The duration of attacks of pain afforded no help in diagnosis.

Frequency and periodicity. In most children the frequency was variable. Pain might occur in single episodes with intervals of weeks; but occasionally many bouts were reported within a period of a few days, with long intervals between. In some instances the increased frequency coincided with the commencement of a new school term, or an examination, attendance at hospital, or some disturbing circumstance at home. In the majority of those children who were admitted to hospital for observation and investigation the pain failed to recur, or attacks were greatly reduced in number, during their stay in hospital.

An attempt was made to separate out a group of children in whom some periodicity in the occurrence of pain was evident. In twenty of a hundred cases pain occurred more or less regularly at intervals of a few weeks or months. In these children vomiting was a common accompaniment, headache might also occur, and in a quarter the temperature was said usually to be raised. Even in this group no increased incidence of organic disease was demonstrated.

---

* It has been claimed that pain persisting for a day or more is indicative of duodenal ulcer, but this has not been confirmed in my original series or subsequently.

ASSOCIATED PHENOMENA

Diarrhoea. In four among a hundred children the stools were said to be consistently 'loose' during attacks of pain, and in eight to be slightly or occasionally so (see page 73, under laxatives).

Vomiting. Nearly two-thirds of the children had a history of vomiting in association with abdominal pain. In most of these it occurred only occasionally, but in one-fifth of all cases it was marked and usual. Nausea was pronounced in nearly half of all cases.

Headache. In one-fifth of cases moderate or severe headache (nearly always generalized) was a feature of the attacks. Between attacks headache occurred in one-quarter, limb pains in 10 per cent, and both headache and limb pains in 7 per cent.

Raised temperature. In five children the temperature was consistently raised during attacks; in an additional six it was raised only once, or occasionally; and in a few the mother thought the child was feverish though the temperature had not been taken.

Pallor. Definite pallor in association with attacks of pain was described in half the cases. In the remainder there was no pallor, or its occurrence was doubtful or occasional. A small number appeared flushed with attacks.

Sleepiness after attacks. In one-quarter of the total number the child was sleepy after bouts of pain. In a few more sleepiness was doubtful or occasional.

Because of the suggested possibility that some of these phenomena are manifestations of *epilepsy*, a special scrutiny was carried out from this point of view. Fits, 'blank spells', 'faint turns', dizziness, and the like were no commoner in children with recurrent abdominal pain than in those without. Moreover, in children with pain the proportion of *epileptiform E.E.G.s* did not vary appreciably according to the character, severity or time of occurrence of the pains. Nor was the proportion of epileptiform E.E.G.s affected appreciably when the children with pain were grouped according to the occurrence or absence of marked vomiting, severe headache, pyrexia or pallor, with attacks, sleepiness afterwards or periodicity of attacks. (See also pages 39 and 88.)

I add two further observations made since the original series was reported.

Smell. In rare instances a peculiar smell may be noticed during an attack, particularly when vomiting is persistent (cyclical vomiting). Investigations so far have not explained it.

Pupil size. I have known three mothers who showed their powers of observation by commenting on the dilated pupils of their child during an attack of pain, or at other times, though they might say 'His eyes were as large as saucers'. This occurrence has not been studied systematically for fear that parents might have new fears put into their minds, but it may be related with the measurement of pupil size discussed on page 99.

Summary

The incidence of recurrent abdominal pain in unselected children was found to be 9.5 per cent in boys and 12.3 per cent in girls (more than a quarter of all girls aged 9 were affected). Differences between the two sexes, as regards incidence and age at onset, appeared from 8 years onwards.

The characteristics of the pain were studied in detail. They afforded little help in diagnosis, though peripheral abdominal pain was rather more likely to be associated with organic disease than was the much commoner central pain.

Other phenomena, such as vomiting, headache, pyrexia, pallor and sleepiness were frequently associated with abdominal pain. Even when they occurred, no correlation with underlying organic disorder or epilepsy could be established.

Chapter 5
Investigation of Organic Abnormalities

Organic diseases. Doubtfully causative and incidental anomalies

The *clinical examination* carried out in the School Series and the School Controls provided data on which to base comparisons. In only two respects, both minor, was a clear difference between the two groups found.

First, in younger children, the average weight of those with recurrent abdominal pain was lower than that of controls by between 1 and 2 lb (0.45 and 0.9 kg); in older children no such difference was found. Second, abdominal tenderness was elicited in more of the children with recurrent abdominal pain than in the controls.

A detailed comparison of such items as height, physique, colouring, condition of the teeth and tongue, palpable lymph nodes and all other abnormalities found on routine examination revealed no significant differences. Minor abnormalities such as lordosis and ectopia testis, occurring slightly more frequently among children with recurrent abdominal pain, will be discussed with the data from the Hospital Series, which will be considered in detail.

The *investigations* carried out in the Hospital Series are tabulated (Table 6). Those cases in which abdominal pain seemed clearly to be due to an organic disorder are summarized (Table 7 et seq.). An organic disorder was accepted as causative if it provided a reasonable basis for the symptoms and, in most cases, if symptoms ceased with appropriate treatment. Borderline cases and incidental anomalies are also summarized and are discussed, because in several instances it was difficult to decide whether the abnormalities found were truly pathological and causative.

ORGANIC CAUSES

In eight cases among a hundred extensively investigated an organic cause for recurrent pain was diagnosed.* (Other causes are discussed in Chapters 8 and 9.)

Table 6. Ancillary investigations. Hospital series (100 children)

Procedure	No. of cases
Mantoux test	88
Urine examination:	
Chemical and microscopic	100
Porphyrins	25
Stool examination or rectal smear:	
For ova and parasites	20
Smear for eosinophils	5
Blood examination:	
E.S.R.	25
White cell count	62
Haemoglobin	35
Glucose tolerance curve	46
Radiological examination:	
Chest	85
Abdomen (plain film)	85
Barium meal and follow-through	25
Barium enema	3
Pyelogram	35
Cholecystogram	4
Electroencephalogram	93
Other investigations:	
Brucella agglutination	20
Brucella agglutination repeated after skin	
(brucellin) test	10
Liver function tests	10

* In a further hundred consecutive cases investigated subsequently the following six causative organic disorders were diagnosed: Urogenital 3 (hydronephrosis 1, persistent renal infection 2), Alimentary 3 (duodenal ulcer 2, gall-stones 1).

In many hundred cases subsequently the percentage of organic disorders accepted as causative has been of the same order.

Table 7. Organic disorders causing recurrent abdominal pain. Hospital series (100 children investigated)

Urogenital:	
Vulvo-vaginitis	1
Urethral cyst	1
Hydronephrosis	1
Recurrent renal infections	1
Alimentary:	
Duodenal ulcer	1
Meckel's diverticulum	1
Calcification of pancreas	1
Colon displacement	1

Urogenital system

JUNE O. *A girl with the common type of central umbilical pain. Chronic vulvo-vaginitis was present but had been overlooked until pus cells were found in the urine. The pains ceased with treatment.*

KATRINA B. *In this girl, with attacks of severe, central, lower abdominal pain, pus cells were found on urine examination. A pyelogram was normal, but endoscopy revealed a urethral cyst. It was removed and the attacks of pain ceased.*

MICHAEL C. *A boy with attacks of pain referred to the umbilicus and also to the left loin. The urine contained pus cells. A pyelogram showed left hydronephrosis; at laparotomy it was found to be associated with a stricture of the upper end of the ureter. After operation attacks of pain ceased.*

MARION C. *A girl aged 7 who in 6 months had had three attacks of pain, mainly in the loins but also umbilical. During attacks there was some frequency of micturition, headache and fever. White cells were found repeatedly in the urine, and B. proteus was grown on culture. A pyelogram and other investigations were negative. She improved with chemotherapy.*

Alimentary system

ROBERT P. *A boy of 9 years, with attacks of epigastric and sub-*

sternal pain. Clear evidence of a duodenal ulcer was obtained on repeated radiological examinations.

MARY F. *In this girl, with central and upper abdominal pain, blood was found in the stools, and pylorospasm was demonstrated radiologically. At exploratory laparotomy a Meckel's diverticulum was found and removed, and the pylorospasm and pain subsequently ceased.*

ROSINA K. *A girl with recurrent pain, probably central, which started unusually early (at a few months of age), and was increasing in severity. At 3 years of age growth was markedly retarded. Radiography showed diffuse calcification of the pancreas, which increased in density during 2 years under observation while the pain became less frequent and less severe.*

CHRISTOPHER D. *A boy with attacks of increasingly severe and frequent widespread abdominal pain, which were associated with gross abdominal distension. A plain radiograph of the abdomen taken during an attack showed extreme dilation of the proximal colon, part of which was interposed between the liver and diaphragm (Chilaiditi's syndrome). Between attacks no physical or radiological abnormality was demonstrated on repeated investigation, though on later re-investigation for melaena a hiatus hernia had become evident. A repair operation was carried out, and the pain and abdominal distension improved. The hiatus hernia subsequently gave rise to complications.*

DOUBTFULLY CAUSATIVE AND INCIDENTAL ANOMALIES

Pain in children with a preceding abdominal disorder

In two children abdominal pain had recurred since an attack of bacillary dysentery, and in two others since an attack of infective hepatitis. In a fifth child pain recurred for 3 years after appendicectomy for acute appendicitis, though there was no previous history of pain. Thorough investigation, however, revealed no evidence of any alimentary, hepatic or other organic disorder. In these five cases there was also positive evidence of an emotional disturbance. It was concluded that the pains were psychologically determined, 'a prolongation of symptoms of an organic disease long past and done with' (Tegner, 1955). With explanation and reassurance the attacks of pain ceased.

Table 8. Doubtfully causative and incidental anomalies. Hospital series (100 children)

	(a) *On clinical examination*		(b) *On investigation*	
Urogenital	Ectopia testis	3	Pyuria	2
			Duplex kidney	1
Alimentary	Defective teeth	—	Aerophagy	2
	Hernia of linea alba	1	Intestinal 'hurry'*	2
	Splenomegaly	1	Duodenal spasm	3
	Rectal fissure	1	Redundant colon	1
			Calcified nodes	3
Skeletal	Marked lordosis	2	Pelvic enchondroma	1
Haematological			Lymphocytosis	1
			Leucocytosis	4
			Leucopenia	5
E.E.G.			Epileptiform	19

* (For discussion on 'irritable colon' see p. 76.)

Other abnormalities found

Abnormalities found on examination or investigation, but not accepted as causing abdominal pain, are summarized (Table 8) and call for discussion.

Urogenital system

Ectopia testis. In three boys with recurrent central abdominal pain, ectopia testis was present.

In the first, both testes were ectopic; in the second, one testis was ectopic and the other lodged at the upper end of the inguinal canal; in the third, one testis was ectopic and associated with a hernia. In the first case the pains ceased without treatment; in the second, pains diminished over a period of several years; in the third the pains ceased after a remedial operation.

In another boy, not in the present series, operation for ectopia testis was followed by relief of long recurrent abdominal pain; but it was instructive to learn that his brother also had recurrent abdominal pain, though normally situated testes, and their mother complained of lifelong attacks of abdominal pain.

Though no similar cases were found among the control series I am averse to including ectopia testis among the immediate causes of recurrent abdominal pains. Admittedly, it is likely that a testis in an abnormal position is more liable than is a normally situated testis to repeated mild trauma, or to torsion resulting in pain; and I have found that among eleven boys with ectopia testis (including three in the present series) five complained of attacks of abdominal pain. It seems unlikely, however, that pain due to such episodes would recur over a period of years.

The loss of pain with simple reassurance suggests one of two possibilities. Either the pain was unrelated to the ectopic testis; or the pain may originally have been provoked by mild trauma of the ectopic testis, and continued subsequently because attention had been focused on the abdomen. On the whole, I subscribe to the latter view, which makes the pains in these boys analogous to those following other abdominal disorders (p. 33) which have resolved. This explanation would account for the different incidence of ectopia testis in the groups with and without pains respectively.

Renal infection. In two children among the series pyuria was found, but only on a single occasion. Pain recurred after the pyuria cleared up, and no other evidence of renal abnormality was found on investigation. Pyuria was considered to have been an incidental occurrence, not related to the symptoms.

Duplex kidney. In this case no evidence of dysfunction or infection was found. Congenital anomalies of the renal tract are not infrequently demonstrated as incidental findings (Bigler, 1929), and this case was considered to be one such example.

Alimentary system

Defective teeth. It is obviously difficult to assess the effect on digestion of one, a few, or even a large number of carious or absent teeth. I was at first impressed by the high proportion of defective teeth among children with pains, but a comparison between the School Series and Controls showed a very close similarity. In the children of both groups a little more than a third were classified as having good teeth; in another third three or more teeth were carious or had been extracted; and in the remainder there were one or two carious teeth. A large number of absent or carious teeth may possibly cause digestive disturbances associated with pain, but in the cases in the present series pain was not considered to be due to gross dental faults.

Hernia of the linea alba. A boy of 11, with a small hernia of the linea alba which disappeared on tensing the abdomen, had complained of central abdominal pain on and off since early childhood. The pains tended to occur when he felt 'worked up'. His father had died when the boy was young, and the boy had many stigmata of emotional stress. It was considered that the hernia was not the cause of his pains, though medical attention had been focused on it. Surgical treatment had been refused.

Splenomegaly. In an unstable and 'difficult' girl, whose spleen was barely palpable (and had been palpated very frequently indeed), investigations revealed no disorder of the liver, haemopoietic or reticulo-endothelial systems. Her attacks of umbilical pain were not considered to be due to the spleen.

Anal fissure. In one boy an anal fissure, associated with constipation and painful defaecation, was found. Central abdominal pain recurred, however, after the fissure was healed and the constipation had been relieved.

Aerophagy. In two children attacks of abdominal pain were associated with marked abdominal distension. Thorough investigation revealed no evidence of organic disease, but in both there was evidence of severe emotional disturbance in the child and in the parents. With reassurance after investigation the attacks of pain and distension became less frequent and severe.

ROGER P. *A boy of 5 years, complaining of attacks of severe periumbilical pain with vomiting and pyrexia, at approximately monthly intervals for 2 years. He was a 'difficult' child, with occasional nightmares. A younger sister had recently begun to complain of abdominal pain and vomiting when Roger's attacks came on. The father was 'often on the verge of a nervous breakdown'. The mother had been under treatment for epilepsy for many years.*

During an attack the boy's upper abdomen was seen to be grossly distended, and radiography showed marked gaseous distension of the stomach and, to a lesser extent, of the intestines. All other investigations (including barium meal examination and E.E.G.) were negative.

Intestinal 'hurry'. In two cases, among the many in whom radiography with barium meal examination was carried out, intestinal 'hurry' was reported.

Duodenal spasm. In two children duodenal spasm was shown radiologically on one occasion, but not on a repeated examination, and was considered to be associated with emotional tension.* In another child duodenal spasm was demonstrated repeatedly, but both spasm and pain were relieved after the removal of a Meckel's diverticulum which had bled frequently.

Redundant loop of colon. Among twenty-five children in whom radiography with barium follow-through examination was carried out, one had a redundant loop of colon. There was no evidence of dysfunction, and the pain was not attributed to this anomaly.

Calcified tuberculous mesenteric nodes. In three of eighty-five children with recurrent pain, radiography demonstrated calcified nodes and a Mantoux test was positive.

Following European practice (Strömbeck, 1932), the case has been put forward (Wallis, 1955a) for regarding tuberculous mesenteric lymph nodes, with calcification, as a cause of recurrent abdominal pain in children. Though calcification is generally accepted as indicating the terminal, non-progressive stage of the inflammatory process, it does not occur suddenly and, while it is proceeding, pain may conceivably be provoked.

The cases in which tuberculous lymphadenitis undoubtedly causes abdominal pain should be readily diagnosable (see p. 59), but in the present series the explanation was not accepted, for the following reasons:

1   The incidence of calcified lymph nodes was no higher than in children without pain. In three among eighty-five children with abdominal pain, radiographs showed calcified nodes, as compared with four in a hundred children without pain from the same district and of comparable ages (Sheach, personal communication).

---

*On several occasions duodenal spasm has been observed to relax and disappear, during radiological screening and barium meal examination of a child with recurrent abdominal pain, after the nervous patient has been put at ease.

2   In some of my patients pain had recurred for years after calcified nodes had been demonstrated, without any evidence of active disease or of change in the degree or extent of calcification. Thus, one boy of 15 years, X-rayed again after an interval of 5 years with no manifest change in the nodes, had complained of attacks of pain over a period of 12 years.

3   Children with calcified abdominal nodes were as prone as those without them to emotional disorders which could account for the pain.

It was concluded, therefore, that in this series calcified nodes were only an incidental finding. (Since the original Hospital Series of investigations, calcified abdominal nodes have become rare in childhood, but recurrent abdominal pains remain exceedingly common.)

Skeletal system

In a girl complaining of recurrent abdominal pain, tuberculosis of the lower thoracic spine was diagnosed clinically and confirmed radiologically. She has not, however, been included in the present series because the pain had occurred over a period of less than 3 months.

Lordosis. Two children in the Hospital Series had marked lumbar lordosis, and a comparison between the School Series and controls produced an impression that lordosis and other forms of defective posture were commoner in children with pains. It was considered that these were not causative, but were more likely to be associated with underlying emotional disturbances, as so graphically described by Cameron (1933). (See also p. 80 for spinal causes.)

Haemopoietic system

White-cell changes. The possible role of infection (bacillary or virus) in the aetiology of recurrent abdominal pains will be discussed later (p. 74). In the present series a small proportion of leucocyte variations was found; but they were transient and variable, and nearly always only slight in degree. In a few cases an associated infection, such as pyelitis or tonsillitis, occurred. In cases where leucopenia was found, brucellosis was investigated, with negative results. Since leucocytosis or leucopenia, which might reflect bacillary or virus infections respectively, was of brief duration, it seemed improbable that a relationship could be established with pains which recurred over a period of many months or years.

ELECTROENCEPHALOGRAPHIC ABNORMALITIES

The cases in the present series formed part of the material of a study designed to investigate the possibility of a relationship between recurrent abdominal pain and cerebral dysrhythmia (Apley, Lloyd and Turton, 1956).

Table 9. Incidence of epileptiform tracings

Schoolchildren	*Epileptiform E.E.G.*
97 with recurrent abdominal pain	10%
202 without recurrent abdominal pain	14.5%
Children attending hospital	
93 with recurrent abdominal pain	19%
57 without recurrent abdominal pain	21%

To preclude any possibility of bias, the reports on all E.E.G.s were made without prior knowledge as to whether they were obtained from children with pains or from those without. In the epileptiform group were included all those with characteristic tracings, whether they occurred at rest, or with hyperpnoea or photic stimulation, even if borderline. Table 9 summarizes the proportions of epileptiform and non-epileptiform tracings found.*

There are speculative explanations for the interesting difference in the proportions of epileptiform E.E.G.s, as between the hospital and non-hospital groups; but the findings clearly do not support the notion that the common type of recurrent abdominal pain is a manifestation of epilepsy. Moreover, in two children with a

* There are considerable differences of opinion about the significance of such abnormalities as focal spikes as manifestations of an epileptic disorder. A detailed analysis of the E.E.G. abnormalities found in schoolchildren is therefore given (Table 9a). It will be seen that if all abnormalities are included, even those of doubtful epileptic significance, there is no significant difference between them in the two groups of children.

history of recurrent abdominal pain an attack of pain occurred while the E.E.G. was being recorded, and in both instances the tracing was normal.

It was concluded from this evidence that cerebral dysrhythmia was not established as a factor in the aetiology of recurrent abdominal pain in children without overt epilepsy.

Summary

Among one hundred children investigated, an organic causative disorder was diagnosed in eight (four alimentary and four urogenital). (Later studies have given similar, or a little lower, figures.) On evidence which is discussed, other abnormalities found were considered to be associated or incidental ('false positives') but not causally related to abdominal pain.

Table 9a. E.E.G.s in schoolchildren

E.E.G. record	202 *children without pain*	97 *children with pain*
Normal	74%	74%
Normal but immature for age	9%	12%
Organic abnormality	0.5%	0%
Localized slow activity	0.5%	0%
Focal spikes	1.5%	4%
Epileptiform	14.5%	10%

Papatheophilou *et al.* (1972) have since described E.E.G. abnormalities of the type usually associated with epilepsy in children with recurrent abdominal pain and other disturbances. A follow-up study of 14 after 12 to 14 years and another group of 50 showed that only one had developed epilepsy (see also p. 88). They conclude that '. . . the finding of E.E.G. abnormalities, other than spike and wave, should not be taken as evidence of epilepsy'.

Chapter 6
Investigation of Intelligence and Emotional Status

Intelligence. Personality traits. Expressions of emotional disturbance. Precipitating factors. Environment: home and school. Organic disorder and emotional disturbance

INTELLIGENCE AND EDUCATIONAL ATTAINMENTS

Assessment in the School Series was based on reports by the headmasters and headmistresses, taking into account the children's abilities and progress. On these factors children are allocated to one of the five 'educational streams', designated A to E from the highest to the lowest. Reports on children with recurrent abdominal pain were compared with those on children without pain, since presumably any errors inherent in the method would be equally applicable to both and should not affect the validity of the comparison. Table 10 shows the almost complete identity between the two groups.

Table 10. Intelligence assessment in schoolchildren

Educational stream	Percentage in children	
	Without pain	*With pain*
A	21.2	20.8
B	28.0	28.3
C	32.1	32.5
D	16.3	16.6
E	2.2	1.6

In the Hospital Series the assessment was made from the interviews with children and parents, from the developmental history, and in some cases from reports by school authorities and by educational psychologists. In a sub-group of twenty-five children in the Hospital Series, selected at random, the intelligence quotient was found to be average or slightly above (Lacey, personal communication). In surprisingly few instances did educational attainments appear to have been limited significantly.

PSYCHOLOGICAL AND EMOTIONAL STATUS

Without employing specialized techniques, the general practitioner or paediatrician assesses psychological and emotional disorders by collating evidence from various sources. First, is his general impression of the child; second, observation of the child-parent relationship; and, third, the information from inquiries about the child's attitude and reactions in different circumstances. The method relies largely on intuition and experience, and is often successful, but inherent in it are some potentially serious errors.

Because a general impression may merely reflect the clinician's pre-conceived ideas, in the present study a scrutiny of specific items was made; and, because of the possibility that unsystematized questioning might leave important gaps, the same detailed questionary was used for all cases, whether seen at school or at

Table 11. Personality traits (schoolchildren)

| | Percentage in children | |
	Without pain	With pain
Normal, average, good	80	51
Hostile, anti-social, unreliable	5	5
Aggressive, quarrelsome, jealous	2	6
Passive, negative	5	4
Highly strung, fussy, excitable	4	21
Anxious, timid, apprehensive	4	13

hospital. As an additional check, the observations were compared with those made independently by a psychiatrist on a sub-group of twenty-five children* forming part of the Hospital Series (Lacey) When the data from the School Series and Hospital Series (including the sub-group) were compared, it was found that the correspondence was close.

Personality traits

As part of the assessment the children were grouped according to their personality traits. The comparison between schoolchildren with and without recurrent abdominal pain is summarized in Table 11.

As compared with the controls, significantly more of the children with recurrent abdominal pain were highly strung, fussy, excitable, anxious, timid, or apprehensive. Most gave an impression of over-conscientiousness, as did also many of their parents.

Often they were 'bad mixers', but aggressive behaviour was uncommon, and, as a generalization, the children could be classified as 'indrawn' rather than 'outgoing'.

Some expressions of emotional disturbance

Expressions of emotional disturbance were considerably commoner among children in the School Series than among the controls. Table 12 summarizes some significant differences.

Among undue fears were included only those (of water, the dark, animals and the like) which were excessive or unusually persistent. Among sleep disorders were included nightmares and

Table 12. Expressions of emotional disturbance

| | Percentage in children | |
	Without pain	With pain
Undue fears	10	27
Nocturnal enuresis	8	20
Sleep disorders	18	39
Appetite difficulties	21	37

* Twenty-five children attending hospital for recurrent abdominal pain were compared with twenty-five attending for other reasons. All were given a detailed psychiatric examination, including projection tests, and an intelligence test.

sleep walking. While inquiring about difficulties of appetite, and feeding habits in general, inquiries were also made concerning the quantity of milk drunk. It was found that, contrary to the view that excessive milk-drinking is associated with recurrent abdominal pain, children with pain drank rather less milk than did the controls. The children with pain tended to be much more fussy about what and how much they ate, and their over-anxious parents spent a considerable time in trying to persuade them to eat. In other respects, such as nail-biting and tics, there was little difference between the School Series and School Controls, though in the psychiatrist's sub-group these two features were rather more common.

In a very small proportion of children among the School and Hospital Series all the above-mentioned disturbances occurred, sometimes with others such as vague and variable pain elsewhere than in the abdomen. In the large majority of the children with pain several of the items mentioned occurred together. *It was the combination of factors which was striking and convincing* and, in practice, it was not difficult to group most of the children either as emotionally disturbed or emotionally stable. An example is the following:

JOSEPHINE D. *A girl of 8, with recurrent, colicky, central abdominal pain since the age of 5. During attacks she looked pale and wanted to lie down. They usually occurred in the morning. She disliked school and was nearly at the bottom of her class. The first attack had occurred soon after she started school when, her mother said, 'she quarrelled with her teacher'. She was frightened of many things, often went and sat alone, was disinterested in food, had bad dreams and nightmares, and sniffed perpetually. Her sister complained of severe dysmenorrhoea. The mother, who poured out the history, herself had frequent headaches and was worried that Josephine might follow in the footsteps of an uncle who was in a mental institution.*

Examination and investigations were negative, except that a pyelogram showed a double kidney on both sides. Inquiries were made at school, and explanations and reassurance were given. Her attacks of pain became less frequent and ceased in a few months. She became 'a happier and brighter person', and was placed second instead of thirty-first in her class.

More difficult cases were those in which expressions of emotional disturbance were not obvious, and the children seemed to be stable and well adjusted. In these, repeated consultations might be necessary; the child's, the mother's, or occasionally the teacher's, confidences when a sympathetic relationship had been established might reveal significant underlying disturbances, as several of the following case summaries show clearly.

SUSAN B. *A girl of 10 years, complaining of recurrent attacks of abdominal pain, usually with vomiting, for more than a year. She slept badly and was 'twitchy', had a poor appetite and was a 'bad mixer'. Her mother had died with gastric carcinoma 6 years previously. Physical examination and investigations were negative.*

Her symptoms continued unabated until a casual remark disclosed that the first attack of pain had occurred on the day after the funeral of a classmate. Thereafter, with sympathetic reassurance, she made a good recovery.

Precipitating* factors

In a few children a clear correlation was obtained between the *first* attack of abdominal pain and a particular stress situation. An example was a girl, Anne P., whose first attack occurred when her mother's renal stone was removed; another was Susan B. (see above).

In many children a relationship between *recurrent* attacks and stress situations was evident.

RICHARD A. *A bright and zestful boy of 9 years, with a talented father who pours tremendous energy into his professional work. Richard had complained of attacks of pain for 2 years. The original attack occurred while his mother was driving him to boarding school for the first time. It was so severe that she seriously considered taking him home, but wisely resisted the impulse. Since then pain has recurred, at the same stage of the journey, each time he is taken back to school at the beginning of term. He soon learned that 'it will get*

---

* *Predisposing and precipitating factors.* 'The distinction is arbitrary but convenient, for the precipitating conditions are but the last of a series of influences which in the end bring about the change in the patient's behaviour. Predisposing conditions produce changes in the patient which determine how he reacts to the precipitating conditions' (Davies, 1957).

better as soon as I'm in school with the other boys'. On the one occasion when he was driven to school during the holidays, to collect a cricket bat, no pain occurred.

An increase in the frequency of attacks was often noted to coincide with examinations at school, or the beginning of school terms. No correlation could be established with seasons when colds and sore throats were rife, an observation not consistent with the suggestion which has been made that attacks of abdominal pain may be associated with upper respiratory infections.

Not infrequently the mother could accurately forecast an attack; she might base her opinion on the child's appearance and behaviour or on the imminence of a school examination or similar stress situation.

ROBERT N. *A boy of 6 years, brought to hospital by an anxious mother complaining that he had had occasional abdominal pain for 3 years, becoming much more frequent and severe in the past year. As an infant he had vomited frequently, and weaning had been troublesome. The pain was severe enough to make him cry, and sometimes vomiting developed after 48 hours. She knew he was going to have an attack because 'he became mopey and a different colour' (possibly yellow).*

Examination and investigations (including liver function tests) were negative. In hospital he had only one attack of pain, on returning from the E.E.G. department. Two months after discharge from hospital there was only one complaint: 'He nearly had a pain at the thought of coming to the out-patient clinic'. The mother then volunteered the information that his pains became worse when he started school, which he disliked, and also at the commencement of the school terms.

Parental (usually maternal) illness or operation, the birth of another child in the family, the removal of the family to a new home, or a change of school, were in some cases similarly associated with attacks of pain.

Again, the onset and localization of attacks of pain could apparently be determined by an organic disease with abdominal symptoms, such as bacillary dysentery or infectious hepatitis. Four such post-infective cases occurred in the Hospital Series, in addition to one post-appendicitis case (p. 17).

What appeared to be direct precipitating factors were elicited in one-third of the Hospital Series. This figure is not, however, truly representative, for the proportion of positives increased towards the end of the study. Though I recognized it early, my reluctance to probe into apparently remote psychological details was only gradually overcome. Accordingly, as more time was devoted to this aspect of the problem, the proportion of positive results increased.

Environment: home and school

Beneath the obvious theme of the child's emotional instability, in case after case there was some less obtrusive discord in the home or at school, or surprisingly often in both together. In Chapter 3 the history of parental illness has been outlined; but it is equally important to consider the attitude of mind in the parents. Assessment is, unfortunately, hardly susceptible to measurement; but among the most consistent impressions from a large number of consultations was that of 'over-protection' of children by excessively anxious parents. In the School and Hospital Series the impression was formed and confirmed repeatedly; in the psychiatrist's sub-group this attitude was apparent in nineteen of twenty-five cases—a proportion nearly two and a half times as high as in children with other complaints. In one or both parents there was an intensive, and sometimes almost obsessional, preoccupation with the child's state of health, reactions and progress.

TERENCE D. *A boy of 11 years, with umbilical pain recurring for a year, sometimes accompanied by scapular and spinal pain, nausea (occasional vomiting) and fever. Mother thought he had had haematemeses, but this had never been confirmed. He had a poor appetite, was moody, had temper tantrums, and sometimes ran away from school.*

The father had always had a stammer. The mother was very obviously domineering and over-anxious, and had no insight into the impressionistic picture she drew during consultations. She continually stressed how much she did for the boy.

According to her story, she had to have an operation before she could conceive, and the parents had to wait 5 years after their marriage before the boy was born. She spent the last month of pregnancy in hospital with haemorrhages, the labour was prolonged, and the baby was jaundiced for several days after birth. There were feeding difficulties from birth—'he gained no weight for the first 6 months and had practically no sleep'. He 'refused to be weaned' and was fed on condensed milk and slops until nearly 2 years of age. (These and other details were gradually obtained during repeated interviews, with the help of a psychiatric social worker who visited the home.) By the age of 4 years a pattern of difficult feeding had been firmly established, with mother spending most of her time 'trying to build him up'.

He started at school when 5 years of age, and often ran home in the first few weeks. There were subsequently frequent absences because of trivial disorders such as colds, and he was behindhand in scholastic progress. The attacks of pain started after he went to a secondary school; he was made a monitor but resigned the post because he lacked confidence.

Thorough physical investigation was negative, with one exception. Barium meal showed considerable delay at the pylorus, due to pylorospasm; when this passed off no abnormalities were seen. He vomited after returning from the E.E.G. department.

Some time after discharge from hospital, when he was said to be somewhat improved, the following dialogue was recorded:

T.D. *'Dad has the same pains as me.'*

Doctor. *'Do you both worry about it?'*

T.D. *'We don't—but Mum puts us to bed all the same.'*

TERENCE R. *A boy of 10 years, complaining of recurrent jabbing, umbilical pain at intervals for many months. On one occasion, though he had passed the preliminary test, he missed the final scholarship examination because of an attack of pain.*

He was said to be afraid to 'venture off' with other boys, or to go into the playground with them. He was a 'picky eater'.

The father had complained of abdominal pains for 14 years. The mother had 'butterflies in the stomach' when she had to face a new contact (this information came out at the second consultation).

Mother had regularly taken him to the near-by school, and brought him home again, until he was 9 years old. His main diet for years, she said, had been Weetabix, and Cow and Gate rice pudding.

Examination and investigations showed no physical abnormality. With simple reassurance he improved rapidly. After 1 month he had

had only one mild pain, was brighter and keener, 'doesn't want Mum with him all the time', 'and goes off with the boys'. Several months later he was very well, full of energy, eating better, and had had no further attacks of pain.

In some instances the disturbance in the child was clearly associated with domestic difficulties. In a few cases there was a strong suggestion of inter-parental tension, a clue which could not be followed in the School or Hospital Series though it was often confirmed in the psychiatrists' sub-group. In this sub-group an undue frequency of financial and housing difficulties, and of sibling rivalry, was also found.

CAROL P. *A girl of 10 years. She had suffered from 'tummy turns all her life', i.e. nausea and pallor for a day every few months. In the past year they had become more frequent, and were associated with central abdominal pain. Headaches occurred either with the attacks or independently.*

The brother of 16 complained of similar episodes. The mother had a tendency to abdominal pain and sickness.

The father was a commercial traveller, and was away from home most of the time. Carol was extremely fond of him: 'When he comes home she gets terribly excited, jumps at him and laughs and cries at the same time.' The mother had not related the attacks to these occasions.

No physical abnormalities were found in this plump girl who faced me with an air of exquisite martyrdom.

At the second consultation mother confessed that she had begun to think that Carol 'worries herself into her pains'. She said that Carol 'got worked up', to a hysterical pitch sometimes, especially when father came home, and might then complain of pain. If she was bothered at school she might get a headache or abdominal pain.

At the third interview Carol was reported to be much improved. Pain had recurred only twice: once when she was about to sing solo at church, and again when she was about to sit an examination in scripture.

JOHN W. *A 6-year-old boy, with recurrent peri-umbilical pain for 3 years. At first attacks occurred every few months; on each occasion he looked ill and stopped playing. Recently they had become more severe; he 'shrieked with agony', vomited and his temperature was raised.*

(Later the mother volunteered the information that the attacks became worse after her charwoman suggested that the cause was 'a twisted gut'.) For weeks before a party he was excited at the prospect, and might become too ill to go when the time came.

The parents had been 'desperately anxious to have a baby', but John was not born until 6 years after the marriage. The labour was difficult (forceps delivery), the baby's face was scratched, and he was difficult to feed. He vomited frequently until weaned on to solids, and after that continued to be difficult with feeding. His temperature was frequently raised (up to 101° F, 38.5° C) for no apparent reason, and the mother said: 'I am always taking it, even though I know most people wouldn't.' He was a nervous boy, who had suffered agonies on going to school for the first time; he was over-conscientious, tried too hard at school, and fussed over trifles. The grandmother, who lived with the family, always had aches and pains, and John was very worried about her.

The father, who had recovered from ulcerative colitis, was serving in the Royal Air Force and was away from home more often than not. Mother had 'doubling up' pains at adolescence. She insisted that she could not disguise her anxiety about her absent husband, her ailing mother, her isolation in the country 'away from everybody', and her highly strung only child.

No physical abnormalities were found on examination and investigation of this boy, whose intelligence and physique were outstandingly good. All treatment proved ineffective.

The child's progress at school was frequently foremost among the parents' preoccupations. Their concern with his position in class, and the results of examinations, often assumed enormous proportions. The child's difficulties at school were only occasionally associated with a lack of ability.

KENNETH B. *A boy of 9 years. He complained of attacks of central abdominal pain for a year, with intervals of 6 weeks, later shortening to 2 weeks. The pain was accompanied by pallor and vomiting, and followed by sleepiness. Examination and investigation (including E.E.G.) were negative.*

At the second consultation further information was forthcoming. It was learnt that the father 'is a great worrier over trifles', and had some abdominal trouble when he returned home after being a Japanese prisoner of war. At first the possibility of school difficulties had been discounted, because Kenneth quite certainly liked going to school and was fond of his classmates and teachers. On closer questioning, however, it appeared that he had considerable difficulty with reading, which worried and upset him. Mother tentatively volunteered that reading lessons made him compare himself with his friends, who read and spelt more easily than he, and that after these lessons pain would develop. Similarly, he might have a pain after an interview with the headmaster to assess his progress.

Inquiries were made at the school, and the headmaster reported that Kenneth was 'conscientious and a hard trier'. After the situation was discussed and adjustments were made the symptoms improved markedly.

More often recurrent abdominal pain and related symptoms were associated with difficulty in establishing satisfactory relations with other children or with teachers.

IAN P. *An only child, 9 years old, complaining of burning (central or epigastric) pain at intervals for 2 years. Attacks usually occurred early in the morning or during school, but never at week-ends or during holidays. Recently they had been associated with vomiting and pyrexia.*

The parents said he was highly strung, lacked self-confidence, and was very critical of himself. He objected to going to school originally, and continued to cry a great deal during the first week of each term.

He was a small, thin, tense boy, easily worried and upset by details or unimportant decisions, such as whether to take off his pullover when he felt hot. His finger-nails were bitten almost to the quick.

Mother was tense and voluble, and admitted to abdominal pains when she was worried. Visited at home, father pooh-poohed the mother's story, and made light of her complaints.

All investigations were negative except that photic stimulation evoked epileptiform characteristics in the E.E.G.

While in hospital for investigation he found it difficult to make friends with other children. He had two mild episodes of pain, which were quickly forgotten when his attention was distracted. On one occasion he admitted that it was worth while being in hospital to avoid having to go to school.

With no treatment other than reassurance and discussion he made

*steady progress. The attacks of pain ceased, and his gain in confidence
was noted in the school report.*

The next case is rather simpler.

ALAN G. *A boy of 9 years, with a 2 years' history of abdominal
pain, recurring every week, often associated with nausea and sometimes with headache. All investigations were negative. On one
occasion in hospital he spontaneously told a nurse that he often
complained of pain to his mother as he found that by doing so he
could avoid going to school. He said that 'the masters are bossy' and
'even smack me' at times.*

Organic disorder and emotional disturbance

Just as an organic disorder may present in a child who is emotionally disturbed, so may emotional disturbance be superimposed
on organic disorder. In a proportion of the children in the
Hospital Series with an organic disorder there was some evidence
of emotional disturbance. Diagnosis was correspondingly difficult
in these cases, but from Table 13 it can be seen that positive or
negative evidence of emotional disturbance is important in attempting to differentiate between organic and non-organic causes of pain.

A further help in differentiation was the fact that nearly half the
children without organic disease had a positive family history of
abdominal pain (p. 14), while in children with organic disease the
proportion was low (1 in 8). Again, in children without organic
disorder a high frequency of precipitating factors, and of an
association between attacks of pain and stress situations, was found.

Table 13 includes an outstandingly interesting group of
thirteen children (four with a family history of abdominal pain).
In this group neither organic disease nor emotional disturbance
could be diagnosed by the methods employed. I was particularly
interested to find out what happened to these children, because of
the possibility that evidence of underlying organic disease or
emotional disturbance might later come to light. In the event, with
explanation and reassurance (after examination and investigation)
the results were excellent. Attacks of pain ceased forthwith in five
cases and soon in the remainder. When inquiries were made
between 1 and 2 years later, information was obtained about most
of the cases and no further attacks had occurred. From this evi-

dence it may be inferred that in some, if not all, of this group an awareness of pain had been acquired by otherwise healthy children (see under Pathogenesis, chap. 9, p. 83).

Table 13. Relation between organic disorder and emotional disturbance. Hospital Series

Emotional disturbance	No organic disorder	Causative organic disorder present
Positive evidence	56	1*
Doubtful evidence	11	2
Negative evidence	13	4
Insufficient data	12	1
	92	8

* Patient with duodenal ulcer (p. 32).

In most cases, however, an accurate diagnosis could be made without delay when all the data of family and personal history, together with the results of clinical and ancillary examinations, were taken into account.

Summary

A comparison of the intelligence of groups of children, respectively with and without recurrent abdominal pain, showed almost complete identity.

As compared with controls, children with recurrent abdominal pain tended to show characteristic personality traits. Expressions of emotional disturbance were considerably commoner, and a combination of these items was usually evident in the individual child. Precipitating factors for the attacks of pain were elicited in one-third of the children.

Chapter 7
Assessment of Treatment

Drug treatment: phenobarbitone, placebo. Therapeutic trial.
Response without drugs. Informal psychotherapy: methods and
results

The results of treatment in children among the Hospital Series
with a causative organic lesion have been summarized (pp. 32–3).
The following remarks refer to children in whom no organic cause
for abdominal pain was found.

The difficulties of attempting to assess and compare the results of
different treatments are considerable, and a complete picture
cannot be drawn if it is to include only those features which lend
themselves to statistical evaluation. Among the difficulties
encountered in these studies were the following: *First*, that the
direct effects of drug therapy could not easily be dissociated from
those of suggestion. *Second*, that I found myself unable to
follow many precedents, by accepting the relief of what is only a
symptom (abdominal pain) as adequate evidence of 'cure'. *Third*,
that estimations of improvement in general well-being remained a
matter for personal judgment, however firm the attempt to base
them on factual reports. *Fourth*, that my views as to the best method
of treatment, and consequently my management of the patients,
became modified during the course of the original studies. In the
following presentation I have tried to overcome these difficulties as
objectively as possible.

DRUG TREATMENT

Often, in practice, the sole treatment offered is a prescription; but,
though claims have been made for a large number of drugs, I
have been unable to find a report of any controlled study. Doubts
about the efficacy of drug therapy are reinforced by cases like the
following:

NORMA S. *A girl of 11 years, complaining of attacks of abdominal pain every week or two for 4 years, was admitted to hospital for investigation. Physical examination and investigations were negative. She was discharged home and phenobarbitone prescribed. Seen as an out-patient 2 months later, she reported that the attacks had ceased. Only when the prescription for phenobarbitone was about to be repeated did the mother confess that, in her pleasure at learning that her daughter had no serious illness, she had forgotten to give any of the tablets. The prescription was torn up. The pain did not return.*

Phenobarbitone. In twenty-four consecutive cases treated with phenobarbitone, the short-term response as regards attacks of pain was as follows. In two-thirds marked improvement or complete relief was noted; among the remaining one-third, in half some improvement was reported with an increase to large doses, while the rest did not improve or became worse. But, among those who had improved, while phenobarbitone was still being taken attacks of pain recurred in six children within a few weeks, and in several more within a few months.

Placebo. In a number of children, chosen at random, sodium citrate tablets were prescribed as a placebo without informing the parents or child. In six children who had lost their pains while taking phenobarbitone, freedom from attacks persisted when the placebo was substituted. In five others, in whom phenobarbitone had failed, or had been only partially successful, attacks of pain ceased when the placebo was given. The following is an example:

ROBERT D. *A 6-year-old boy, with a history of attacks of pain for 3 years. E.E.G. was characteristic of epilepsy. Physical examination and other investigations were negative. On phenobarbitone there was considerable improvement for 3 months. Attacks of pain then became more severe and frequent and the placebo was substituted. He promptly lost his pains, and the attacks failed to recur for 2 years (when he was last seen) after all treatment had ceased.*

In some cases sodium citrate was prescribed as the first form of drug therapy, and usually the attacks of pain were relieved.

Therapeutic trial
In a series of thirty-six children attending an out-patient clinic

with recurrent abdominal pain, a simple therapeutic trial was carried out. Either phenobarbitone or sodium citrate was dispensed; after a period of 1 to 2 months the other drug was substituted. Neither the patient nor the parents, nor I as the clinician, knew which of the two drugs was given. During this trial only a minimum of explanation was offered. After a period of several months, and only after the effects of therapy had been assessed, the identity of the drug used in each case was disclosed to me for the first time.

Four of the children (two taking phenobarbitone and two taking the placebo) who lost their pain developed other complaints (dizzy feelings in one, headaches in two, and a tic in the fourth).

It was found that in the group as a whole no definite differences had been established between the therapeutic effects of phenobarbitone and sodium citrate.

Other drugs

In a small number of cases not included in the present series phenytoin or troxidone was prescribed, and in a few others 'Oblivon' (methylpentynol). Some children were given 'old-fashioned' mixtures containing belladonna, or rhubarb and gentian, or agar. The conclusion reached was that any or all of these drugs might seem effective, but the effects were variable, unpredictable and often transient.

Ergotamine is ineffective (Graham, 1969) and neither anti-cholinergic nor anti-spasmodic drugs are of value (Illingworth, 1971).

It has been claimed that anti-depressant drugs are effective (Frommer, 1967) and when depressive-illness is diagnosed in a child with recurrent pains it is reasonable to give such drugs as one part of comprehensive treatment for this rare condition in childhood.

No drugs

In many children a marked improvement was observed without the use of any drugs. During the period when phenobarbitone was prescribed for twenty-four children (p. 55) a further twenty were treated without sedation or any form of drug therapy (the number was subsequently increased considerably). I was not able to satisfy myself that there was an appreciable difference in the short-term response between the two groups, except that children on drug therapy were more likely to develop 'substitution symptoms' (see above). The long-term response will be discussed later.

In many cases it was observed that attacks of pain occurred much less frequently or, in the majority, ceased completely, while the children were in hospital for investigation without treatment, though attacks of pain might recur later. A similar improvement was common in children investigated as out-patients. The effect seemed to be enhanced, and was often quite dramatic, if the purpose of the investigations was made clear while they were being carried out, and if the exclusion of organic disease was confidently explained to the parents.

A similar dramatic improvement sometimes occurred in children after operation. If the operation was appendicectomy the 'cure' might be attributed to it, even if the appendix was healthy; but a similar improvement was occasionally observed after tonsillectomy or other operation.

From the above observations and the results of the therapeutic trial described it was inferred that drugs play a very subsidiary part in the treatment of children with recurrent abdominal pain; and that investigations and hospitalization, with or without operation, may be effective because they allay anxiety.

I conclude that in this disorder drugs are rarely more than a vehicle for suggestion therapy. Because reliance on drug therapy implies a superficial approach to the problem, the long-term results are likely to be less satisfactory than those obtained by treatment of the underlying disturbances.

INFORMAL PSYCHOTHERAPY

Quite early in these studies I had to face the problem which Fletcher and Jacobs (1955) put in these words: 'How far into the psychoneurotic aspects is it wise for those of us with limited psychiatric knowledge to go?' Their attitude, that 'this must depend on experience, interest and the time at one's disposal', and their view that one should try the effects of 'simple rationalization', broadly describes my own. The contrary view would have entailed transferring a considerable proportion of routine paediatric cases for formal psychiatric diagnosis and treatment. A popular alternative, to dismiss the patient with the remark that 'there is nothing organically wrong', seems to me to be unethical. Moreover, it might provoke the reply: 'But that nothing hurts.' I preferred what may be called 'informal psychotherapy' (the term 'modified insight therapy' has also been used), but I am still searching for a better term.

Outline of methods

At the first consultation a discussion of symptoms and background was followed by careful physical examination and the necessary minimum of investigations. Usually their purpose and results were explained to the parents at the second consultation, when their fears as to the cause of the symptoms were fully discussed.

The identification of a specific anxiety in the parent's or child's mind might be dramatically effective. It would enable one to say 'He has not got appendicitis' (or leukemia or cancer, or whatever the fear might be). 'He will not have to come into hospital. He will not have to have an operation.' The mere verbalization of fears often seemed to have a beneficial effect. Without the identification of a specific anxiety (which, it is important to remember, might not be elicited at the earliest consultations) reassurance was also effective, as a rule. Reassurance was never given without explanation. To say to parents 'Don't worry' is pointless: as parents they *should* worry if they fear their child is ill, and it is the doctor's task to dispel their fears. To reinforce the reassurance, attention was drawn to encouraging features of the child's history, development and physique. Sympathetic guidance was offered on the lines discussed later (Chap. 10). If further interviews seemed to be indicated it was suggested to the parents that they should try to observe any association between the occurrence of stress situations and pain. Their reaction, at once or at the next consultation, was often one of whole-hearted agreement and relief. When his confidence had been won the child might be seen without his parents. A few children who were not responding satisfactorily were admitted to hospital for further observation.

In some instances, after the first consultations attacks of pain ceased or became milder and less frequent. If attacks persisted or recurred, as they did in a proportion, they were almost always less severe and more readily dealt with by the parents. In this group undue attention to the minutiae of the pain was avoided, as was also repeated examination of the abdomen. Instead, further detailed inquiries into the background were made; for example, a survey of all the circumstances which preceded the attack would be made. Those arising in the home were relatively easy to elicit; but a mother might say that her child 'gets on all right at school' when she herself had not been in or near the school for years, and it was sometimes necessary to exchange information with the teacher.

Results

One child in ten in the Hospital Series was considered to need referring to a psychiatric colleague for advice and treatment. I learned to recognize fairly easily this small minority. Nearly always they came from families in which some other member or members (usually one or both parents) showed evidence of a marked anxiety state, or depressive illness in a small proportion. The whole family might be in need of treatment, and one was at a loss as to which was the patient. In this group treatment was often protracted and the results not very satisfactory.

Treated children: long term follow-up

In the remainder informal psychotherapy was helpful. For non-organic disorders it is often impossible to speak of 'cures'; but in many of the children in this group attacks of pain quickly ceased or improved, in some others improvement occurred more slowly, and relapses were uncommon. Perhaps even more gratifying was the improvement in general attitude and reaction to difficult situations which was evident in many cases (see Josephine D., p. 44, and Terence R., p. 48, as examples).

In order to compare psychologically treated with untreated children more exactly, and over a long period, a follow-up survey in the same geographical area as previously was undertaken (Apley and Hale, 1973). Most of the patients and many parents were interviewed in their homes, not by me but by a colleague. Thirty children (boys and girls in equal numbers) comprised the series, as in the previous one (pages 18–21), and the same criteria for selection were used. The follow-up period was 10 to 14 years when the treated patients (now 15 to 28 years old) were assessed. From the information obtained several questions could be answered.

Do they 'grow out of' pains?

In 19 of 30 treated cases abdominal pains ceased, 14 quickly after treatment was started and five later. In the remaining 11, pains of some degree continued into adolescent or early adult life, which was as far as the survey could be taken. Though these overall figures are far from showing the whole picture, superficially they are almost identical with those of the earlier, untreated series (Table 14).

Table 14. Results of present study compared with earlier series.

No. at follow-up	Previous untreated series	Present treated series
No abdominal pains, no other symptoms	9	9
No abdominal pains, but other symptoms	9	10
Abdominal pains continuing, with other symptoms	12	11

Nevertheless, in those treated cases where the attacks of pain ceased they did so promptly in 14 of 19 treated cases (Table 15), but in only two of 10 untreated cases for whom the information is available. Moreover, once the pains ceased they did not recur later in any treated cases but did recur in four of the untreated ones.

In both series just under a third of the cases became free of all symptoms. Those remaining, who grew up with abdominal pain or other symptoms, will be compared.

What of the severity of the attacks ? In 11 of the treated series attacks of pain persisted into adolescence or early adult life. The attacks of pain at the time of follow-up are summarized in Table 15; in two cases they continued to be severe and frequent.

Table 15. Follow-up of 30 treated cases with abdominal pains

	No. of cases
No pains (rapidly ceased 14, slowly ceased 5)	19
Mild and infrequent	7
Moderate, less frequent	2
Severe and frequent	2

In one of the two severe cases pain was consistently right-sided from the age of 6; at 21 years of age bilateral ovarian cysts were removed and the pains did not recur.* In the other severe case with continuing pain the patient later lost weight and at 17 years a depressive state was diagnosed.

Are they liable to other disorders later?

Table 16 shows what other disorders developed in the 21 patients with continuing symptoms, and makes a comparison with the untreated series. Rather interestingly, there was in this respect little difference between those patients with or without continuing abdominal pains. Treatment appears to have made a small but significant contribution.

Table 16. Follow-up: frequency of non-abdominal disorders

	30 cases untreated	30 cases treated
Number with persisting disturbances	21	21
Migraine	3	0
Headaches (severe or moderate)	15	4
Dysmenorrhoea	5	3
Other pains	1	1
Other bodily symptoms	4	6
'Nerves', anxiety	13	10

Do they live ordinary lives when they grow up?

How the patients 'lived with their symptoms' is shown in Table 17.

In all but the two severe cases the treated patients understood and accepted the association of stress and pain. In all but these two their symptoms did not cause absenteeism from work or interference with their activities. The information in the earlier, untreated series is insufficient for an exact comparison, though we know that three-quarters of those with continuing abdominal pains were not well adjusted. We believe that adaptation, based on an understanding of the disorder, was far from satisfactory in many

* She had been investigated more exhaustively than any other patient, partly because of my guiding rule that the further the pains are from the centre, the more likely are they to be due to organic disease.

Table 17. Follow-up of 21 treated cases

Abdominal Pains	Work and other activities	
	Restricted	Not restricted
None	—	10
Mild or moderate	—	9
Severe and frequent	2	—

of the untreated cases and both their work and other activities suffered more.

The treatment given cannot be claimed to have 'cured' the pains, but it was helpful in speeding the recovery from attacks of pain and in lessening the occurrence of other symptoms, both physical and nervous. It seemed also to increase the patient's adaptability and make it more likely that he could live a normal life. In this follow-up of treated cases, half the patients were interviewed with their parents. Years after treatment was finished these parents emphasized, time and again, the good effects of reassurance with explanations and discussions, both on themselves and on their children. After all, the family is a unit of disease.

Comments

In discussing treatment it has been necessary also to outline the methods of diagnosis, for diagnosis and treatment may be inseparable and continuous processes. I was constantly relearning two lessons. Treatment begins with the first words spoken at the first diagnostic consultation; and the more time is spent on the history, the less time is likely to be needed for treatment.

Summary

Drugs were found to play little, if any, part in the treatment of recurrent abdominal pain in children, except as a vehicle for suggestion. A minor disadvantage of drug therapy is that, even if attacks of pain cease, 'substitution symptoms' may develop. More fundamental is the implication that a symptom, and not the underlying disturbance, is being treated.

A small minority (less than one-tenth) of children attending hospital with the complaint of recurrent abdominal pain were considered to need specialized psychiatric treatment. They came of families in which a parent had disturbances associated with a marked anxiety state or, occasionally, depression.

In the large majority of the remainder treatment by 'informal psychotherapy' was successful, and sometimes dramatically so. The success of treatment was estimated not only by cessation of abdominal pain, but also by an improvement in the children's reactions to difficult situations and by their general well-being.

Part II
Discussion

Chapter 8
Organic Causes

Organic v. non-organic. Classification. Site of the disorder.
Discussion of causes: obstruction, reflex stimulation, miscellaneous

A family doctor's letter, brought to my clinic with a boy complaining of recurrent abdominal pain, concluded with the terse remark: 'Kindly examine the *soma* and leave the *psyche* to me.'

'In the course of the nineteenth century it had become an almost unchallenged axiom that the study of disease could be approached from two completely different points of view: the organic approach, according to which only material causes were recognized as able to produce organic disease, or the psychological attitude, according to which mental processes could produce functional disorders only. Modern psychosomatics has demonstrated that this distinction is not in harmony with the observed facts: emotional processes can produce and influence organic illness, organic disturbances can produce mental disease' (Groen, 1957). Many would go further, 'The word psychosomatic is itself misleading; even though I use it, I distrust it. It tends to perpetuate the illusory duality of mind and body associated with Descartes and his intellectual supermarket. There are no separate minds and bodies—only human beings. As children themselves might do, let me put this in a simple phrase: "*The ill child is ill all over*" ' (Apley, 1973).

It may appear that the separation of organic and non-organic disorders in the present studies has, by the very method of presentation, been given undue emphasis. In children with recurrent abdominal pain the symptom may originate in association with emotional disturbance (presumably mediated through the hypothalamus) or with gross pathological change in an abdominal organ. Whatever the cause, the final common path has been stimulated, and pain is felt. There is, however, an obvious organic element in emotional responses, like blushing; and an obvious element in organic disorders, such as the coeliac syndrome or any structural lesion which is accompanied by pain. The question of 'either . . . or . . . ' is therefore, an over-simplification.

Nevertheless, the differentiation between primarily organic and primarily non-organic disorder remains one of the basic tenets of medical practice. No clinician can afford to overlook the diagnosis of organic lesions, which are often and quickly curable: the penalty for such an oversight may be the child's death. Since the essential of rational treatment is exact diagnosis, the prime disturbance, however confusingly it may be overlaid, should be disentangled from its associations and complications.

On two main grounds, therefore, I justify the attempt at clear separation of organic from non-organic causes. First, that this is a practical method of approach in diagnosis; and, second, that by this means discussion is simplified.

CLASSIFICATION OF CAUSES

Because of the large number and variety of possible causes, and the overlapping between them, no classification is entirely satisfactory. From the clinician's point of view a simplified topographical grouping has advantages. The history, examination and investigations may indicate:

(a) *Intra-abdominal disorder* (intestine, renal tract, other structures).
(b) *Disorder of surrounding parts* (spine, thorax, pelvis, genitalia).
(c) *Disorder of nervous system* (tumour, encephalitis, epilepsy, emotional disturbance).
(d) *Generalized disorder* (infective, allergic, metabolic, toxic).

For the purpose of discussion, however, possible causes of recurrent abdominal pain are grouped under the headings of Obstruction, Reflex Stimulation and Miscellaneous and are considered in this and the subsequent chapter.

Such disorders as paroxysmal tachycardia or asthma, in which attacks may be associated with abdominal pain, should be borne in mind but have been excluded here. I quote only one example.

ROGER B., *aged 7, was admitted to hospital for 'appendicitis' with several years history of bouts of abdominal pain. He had tachycardia of 280 a minute and pain was localized to the liver, which was tender because of cardiac failure. His mother remarked: 'The attacks upset him so much that I can see his heart beating nineteen to the dozen through his clothes'!*

I. Obstruction
Intestinal stenosis at different levels, pylonic stenosis, hernia, diverticulum, superior mesenteric artery syndrome, recurrent intussusception or volvulus (possibly with malrotation), regional ileitis, polyp, neoplasm; adhesions or other inflammatory processes; foreign bodies, worms, constipation (simple or associated with anal fissure, megacolon, fibrocystic or coeliac disease). Renal, biliary and pancreatic colic: pseudo-colic.

II. Reflex stimulation
Infection (e.g. appendicitis, cholecystitis, hepatitis, dysentery), irritable colon syndrome, sterile inflammation (periodic peritonitis), toxocariasis, adenitis (tuberculous, non-specific, neoplastic), sickle cell disease, ovulation, torsion of gonads, peptic ulcer, excessive air-swallowing.

III. Miscellaneous
Spinal disease, allergic disorder, hereditary angioneurotic oedema, metabolic disorder (hypoglycaemia, diabetes mellitus, porphyria, hyperbilirubinaemia, hyperlipaemia), lead poisoning, abdominal migraine or epilepsy, emotional disorders.

Site of the disorder
In the attempt to eliminate or confirm among the embarrassingly large number of possibilities, localization of the site of the disorder may first be considered.

In theory, though not always in practice, the area on the surface to which visceral pain is referred indicates the site of the disorder, as summarized thus:

Site of referred pain	Site of disorder
Epigastrium	Stomach
Umbilicus	Small intestine

Supra-pubic area	Ascending colon
Deep pelvis	Sigmoid colon
R. upper abdomen	Liver and gall-bladder
Loin and groin	Kidney and ureter

In the large majority of cases the child points to or round the umbilicus as the site of the pain. The small intestine would accordingly seem an obvious site of the underlying disorder. As far as the evidence goes, however, this suggestion remains unconfirmed. Clinically, evidence of bowel dysfunction is uncommon. Radiological studies, carried out in some of the Hospital Series, between, and occasionally during, attacks of pain, did sometimes demonstrate abnormality of structure or motility. However, at laparotomy, though lymph nodes are often numerous in the mesentery of the terminal ileum (Gross, 1953), manifest disease of the small intestine or the surrounding structures is a rarity.

In practice, therefore, and especially in young children, localization of the pain is unhelpful in the large majority of cases. How-

Table 18. Site of pain in twenty children with organic disorder

	Disorder	*Site*
Urogenital	Vulvo-vaginitis	Umbilical
	Cystine stones R. ureter	Umbilical
	Hydronephrosis (3 cases)	Umbilical and loin
	Hydronephrosis	Loin
	Recurrent renal infection (2 cases)	Loin
	Urethral cyst	Supra-pubic
	Duplex kidney with stones	Supra-pubic
Alimentary	Cholecystitis	Umbilical
	Calcified pancreas	Umbilical
	Meckel's diverticulum	Umbilical and R. iliac fossa
	Cholecystitis	Umbilical and R. hypochondrium
	Meckel's diverticulum	Loin
	Partial duodenal obstruction	Loin
	Colon displacement	Epigastric
	Duodenal ulcer (3 cases)	Epigastric and Substernal

ever, a rule has been evolved which has proved helpful in diagnosis: *The further the localization of the pain from the umbilicus, the more likely is there to be an underlying organic disorder.*

Table 18 summarizes the site of pain in twenty consecutive children (including eight described in the Hospital Series) with recurrent abdominal pain due to an organic disorder. In four the pain was central (umbilical or peri-umbilical); in the remaining sixteen, though the umbilicus was also involved in five, the pain was consistently felt in the periphery of the abdomen.

I. Obstruction

Mechanical obstruction was demonstrated in only one of the one hundred cases in the Hospital Series (Chilaiditi's syndrome). In other published series the proportion has also been very small. Nevertheless, the possible causes must always be considered.

Congenital anomalies. It is recognized that congenital anomalies of the alimentary tract may not produce symptoms from birth, and when symptoms eventually develop they may be intermittent. Examples are malrotation or mild stenosis of the intestine. A common symptom is vomiting, and if the patient is examined during an attack abdominal distension is generally seen. This sign should suggest confirmation by plain radiographs during an attack, and barium studies between attacks. Abdominal distension may, however, occur with excessive air-swallowing alone.

Congenital hypertrophic pyloric stenosis (sequelae). A recent report (Dodge, 1974) on sequelae of pyloric stenosis is of great interest. 360 patients who had been operated on were followed up 1 to 18 years later and 56 were found to complain of recurrent abdominal pain. 17 of these were X-rayed, of whom 7 had duodenal ulcers and 1 a gastric ulcer. Other observers have found few or no peptic ulcers on follow-up after operation, though delayed gastric emptying has been reported. The discrepancies are difficult to evaluate.

In the *superior mesenteric artery syndrome* (Hyde *et al.*, 1963) the distal duodenum is compressed by the dorsal mesentery, as may be shown radiologically. The pain is unusual in that it occurs typically after meals and may be relieved in the prone position. I have not seen a definite case; in one boy, in whom the X-ray appearances were suggestive, the pains cleared up without an operation or any other physical treatment.

Crohn's disease (regional enteritis or ileitis) is rare in childhood. The common presentation is persistent or recurrent abdominal pain (usually peri-umbilical) with failure to thrive, weight loss and slight fever. A tender abdominal mass may be felt. Peri-anal disease (fissures or ulceration) may occur with or even before the onset of intestinal disturbances. Oral ulceration tends to be overlooked but may occur at some stage of the disease (Croft and Wilkinson, 1972).

Polyp or neoplasm. A polyp or a neoplasm may be suspected if the child is anaemic, if blood is found in the stool, if the general condition is poor, or, in advanced cases, if a mass is felt abdominally or rectally. Presenting with the single or predominant feature of recurrent abdominal pain, polyp or neoplasm is extremely uncommon.

Adhesions. The history, and confirmatory evidence of inflammatory disease, may suggest this diagnosis, which is, however, only rarely confirmed.

Foreign body, gall stones. The diagnosis of foreign body or gall stones should be suggested by the characteristic history and confirmed radiologically.

Despite older views, only 5 per cent to 10 per cent of children with gallstones prove to have underlying haemolytic disease (Söderland and Zetterström, 1962; Shrand and Ackroyd, 1973). Gallstones or cholecystitis should be suspected if there is a personal or family history of haemolytic disease or liver disease, or a history or signs of obstructive jaundice or pain or tenderness in the right hypochondrium. Even with acceptable grounds for suspicion, cholecystography (see p. 73) confirms the diagnosis only rarely.

Worms. In the past, the bed-pan was a happy hunting ground for theories, as for worms. The role of threadworms or roundworms in the production of abdominal pains is rarely accepted nowadays for, if pains occur, they and the worms may come and go with no apparent inter-relationship. In the Hospital Series worms and ova were looked for in stools and smears from twenty patients, but were found in only one. Wood *et al.* (1955) found a high incidence of thread-worm infection in their cases (13 per cent), but the incidence was slightly higher in their control group of children without pain. In Western countries, as least, it appears highly improbable that worms are responsible for recurrent abdominal pain.

Constipation. Despite the over-simplified pronouncement that constipation never causes symptoms, it may do so. A relatively common cause of what is aptly named 'obstipation' is anal fissure in infants or children (Apley, 1954). In this condition, and in the rarer causes of constipation (e.g. megacolon), the presenting symptom is nearly always the constipation itself or painful defaecation, with which abdominal discomfort may be associated; for this reason no case of anal fissure has been included as a cause of recurrent abdominal pain of long duration. Visual, rather than digital, examination permits a quick and relatively painless diagnosis of fissure. Megacolon and coeliac disease are suggested by the permanently protuberant abdomen and readily confirmed by ancillary investigations. From Table 4 it is seen that simple constipation is, at most, a rare cause of recurrent abdominal pain.

Fibrocystic disease may be associated with abdominal pains, often with palpable faecal masses (Gracey *et al.*, 1969), which can be relieved by oral N-Acetyl cysteine.

In some instances I have considered recurrent abdominal pain might be associated with the taking of *laxatives*, especially in the occasional case (page 28) with loose stools. I have not encountered cases so severe as those described in adults (women) with abdominal pain, diarrhoea, weight loss and electrolyte abnormalities due to excessive taking of laxatives (Cummings *et al.*, 1974).

Renal, biliary and pancreatic colic. Among these varieties of colic the second is very uncommon; the third is extremely rare in childhood, though Nash (1971) has reported familial pancreatitis which can present in childhood with recurrent abdominal pain. Even in children a careful history and examination, especially during an attack of pain, may reveal that the pain is not, or is not exclusively, localized to the centre of the abdomen, but is also referred respectively to the right hypochondrium, or the loin (Table 18). Microscopic examination of the urine is, however, essential in the investigation of all cases; a plain radiograph of the abdomen is helpful in demonstrating calculi, and pyelography or cholecystography is advisable if the clinical indication exists.

Even in the absence of microscopic abnormalities in the urine, if pain is consistently felt in the loin, pyelography is advisable; though even in such cases only a small minority have a demonstrable organic lesion.

JOHN M. *A boy of 10 years (not included in the Hospital Series) with a history of recurrent abdominal pain for 6 years. Five years previously, when the pain was vaguely referred to the centre of the abdomen and did not certainly extend into the left loin, microscopic urine examination had been negative. The pain became milder and occurred very infrequently. At 10 years of age attacks became more severe and frequent, and pain was definitely located in the loin. Again microscopy of the urine was negative, but a pyelogram showed advanced hydronephrosis of the left kidney.*

Pseudo-colic. I have seen several children, usually in their 'teens, with a history of bouts of severe abdominal pain which caused them to writhe and shriek 'in agony'. The previously suggested diagnosis was usually renal colic; but, both in the acute phases and between, investigation of the renal tract was negative in all of them and the children had considerable emotional problems for which treatment was necessary.

II. Reflex stimulation
Inflammation. The evidence of inflammation in these cases may be considered in general, before individual causes are discussed.

In most cases abdominal pain occurs without fever, but in the small proportion (p. 28) in which the temperature is raised, suspicions of an inflammatory cause are especially roused. There is a considerable body of evidence to show that recurrent fever may be associated with emotional disturbance (Mac Keith, 1953), and in children with recurrent abdominal pain evidence of infection is rarely convincing. Thus, leucocytosis, which would be expected in a pyogenic infection, is exceptional. In a few cases, on the contrary, leucopenia is found, which may suggest the possibility of abortus fever or a virus infection. The fever usually disappears quickly, and its course is not appreciably affected by antibiotics or chemotherapy. An alleged association with 'infections in the upper respiratory tract, recurrent exacerbations of which seem to have a trigger effect' has been passed on from one author to another, but 'the direct symptoms and sign may be so slight as to escape notice' (Kempton, 1956); and, indeed, they are rarely convincing except in acute, infrequent episodes. In the School Series there was no evidence that upper respiratory infections were commoner than in controls; nor was an increased incidence of pains apparent at times when upper respiratory infections were prevalent in the community.

Appendicitis. Though appendicectomy in children with recurrent abdominal pains is still relatively frequent, the diagnosis of 'chronic', 'recurrent' or 'grumbling' appendicitis is less common nowadays than it used to be. Nevertheless, the contrary view, that 'the appendix never grumbles; it screams, or remains silent', may be going too far in the opposite direction and equally calls for examination.

Appendicectomy has been performed in many children with a long history of recurrent pains (Chap. 3). Often the operation is done during an acute phase, but obvious inflammation of the appendix is not commonly described, even though the criteria used are variable. Nevertheless, it is obviously important to remember that there is, of course, nothing to prevent acute appendicitis from occurring in the one-tenth of all children who have recurrent abdominal pain, just as it may occur in others.

In a hundred consecutive children with recurrent pain in whom appendicectomy was performed, Fitzsimons (1946) reported a non-inflamed appendix in ninety-four; mild, catarrhal appendicitis in two; and chronic obstructive appendicitis in four. From another series of a hundred operated cases, Stuckey (1950) concluded that: 'Pathologically the condition of subacute or chronic appendicitis is not common, and such terms as used by clinicians are not scientific, except occasionally.' Moreover, in Stuckey's cases there was no evident correlation between loss of symptoms after operation and the pathological findings reported.

Even the pathological evidence cannot be accepted without discussion. Boyd (1947) has written: 'Today every appendix is condemned by some pathologist somewhere.' Acute appendicitis the pathologist knows and understands, but healed appendicitis may easily be interpreted as chronic appendicitis. 'Of the occurrence of "chronic appendicitis", of a continuing low-grade infection with its typical cellular reaction, the pathologist has no experience. If it exists at all it must surely be a rare disease' (*Brit. med. J., 1955*).

The clinical diagnosis of acute appendicitis in children is notoriously fraught with difficulty, and where genuine doubt exists it is clearly safer to operate. Moreover, if the pains continue afterwards, the doctor is comforted by knowing that he is not overlooking a potentially dangerous condition. It seems, however, most unlikely that recurrent or chronic appendicitis can cause *frequent* attacks of pain over a period of many months or years. My practice is to advise against operation unless, during an attack, there is evidence of localization of pain, together with definite tenderness and resistance, in the right iliac fossa. I consider *the crucial feature in diagnosis to be a change in symptomatology* (e.g. case 5, p. 16).

Irritable colon (irritable bowel) syndrome. Stone and Barbero (1970) studied a group of children with recurrent abdominal pain and the expected variety of other somatic and behavioural symptoms and they have proposed that the abdominal manifestations be described as 'The Irritable Bowel Syndrome of Childhood'. The main features prominent in Stone and Barbero's series, as well as my own, include pallor and headache; familial anxiety and precipitation of pain by stress; negative physical, X-ray and laboratory investigations. In addition they described pellet-like stools and tenderness on deep palpation over the colon (though it should be noted that the pains are commonly peri-umbilical), as well as areas of hyperaemia and related changes in the rectal mucosa. The irritable colon syndrome of adults is probably best described as the irritable bowel syndrome (*Lancet*, 1969): pain may be felt anywhere in the bowel but commonly in the left iliac fossa; in adults it is often associated with eating and also with defaecation. It is thought to be provoked by spasm, inco-ordinated or irregular contraction of the intestine, and to be associated with changes in intra-lumenal pressure. Like other recurrent abdominal complaints the irritable bowel syndrome is commonly associated with emotional disturbances: it is either neurotic or psychosomatic (*Lancet*, 1969). Even if irritable colon or bowel could be accepted as a distinct entity in childhood, it seems undesirable to use a label that will misleadingly focus attention on one part of the body. Both for diagnosis and management, is not attention better directed to the whole person ?

Periodic peritonitis. I have not seen any examples of this mysterious condition, described (Reimann *et al.*, 1954) as a cyclical, sterile peritonitis occurring predominantly in Jews, Armenians and Arabs.

Toxocariasis. In a considerable series of children and adults

Garrow and Kane (1973) postulated toxocariasis as a possible cause of epilepsy, asthma, 'growing pains', Henoch-Schonleim purpura and recurrent abdominal pains, in addition to the generally recognized manifestations. The fluorescent antibody test for specific toxocara immunoglobulins was done in 12 of my cases with recurrent abdominal pain; in this small number none proved positive.

Non-specific mesenteric adenitis. The condition of acute non-specific mesenteric lymphadenitis was clarified by Brennemann (1921). He described an acute abdominal condition, in association with an acute throat infection, in which the abdominal symptoms are evidently due to associated mesenteric lymphadenitis. It appears to have been assumed that chronic non-specific mesenteric lymphadenitis may arise in the same way. Alternatively, it has been attributed to an unidentified alimentary infection (possibly virus). The latter possibility gains some support from reports of a degree of inflammation of the terminal ileum in a proportion of operated cases (13 per cent of Fitzsimons's (1946) series). Nevertheless, the evidence for infection is extremely unsatisfactory.

Ward-McQuaid (1951) reviewed 500 children in whom the appendix had been removed for suspected appendicitis or mesenteric adenitis, and reported lymph node enlargement in 17.2 per cent of cases; the proportion was roughly the same both in emergency cases and waiting-list cases, and is surprisingly low when compared with Fitzsimons's (1946) incidence of 100 per cent. What is lacking is a large series of *normal* controls, for it is recognized that large mesenteric lymph nodes are often found incidentally at operation (Gross, 1953), or at necropsy in children after sudden death (Penner, 1949). It is conceivable that adenitis, by irritating the bowel or peritoneum, may provoke pain; but the supposition would gain force if large nodes were proved to be significantly commoner in children with recurrent pains than in those without them.

If the nodes often found at operation are removed, no organisms can be cultured (Ward-McQuaid, 1951) and examination reveals a 'reactive hyperplasia' (but see under Yersinia (page 79)).

My material supports Ward-McQuaid's view that there is not the seasonal variation, nor the increased frequency of cases at times when respiratory infections are prevalent, which would be expected if, for example, respiratory virus infection were the cause of recurrent pains.*

As a final observation on mesenteric adenitis, I have compared the curves for the incidence and onset of recurrent abdominal pain (Figs. 1 and 2) with the curve for normal lymphoid growth (including 'intestinal lymph masses') drawn by Scammon (1930). The lymphoid type of growth continues steadily until about the age of 12 years; the curve shows no similarity with Figs. 1 and 2.

Conway's (1951) statement that 'the conception of chronic non-specific mesenteric adenitis lacks a sound pathological basis' clearly sums up the available evidence.

Other causes of adenitis. In a proportion of the Hospital Series, serological studies (Table 6) were carried out, in view of the possibility that abortus fever might produce lymphadenitis and hence pain. The evidence from these tests was completely negative. Fitzsimons (1946) and others have ruled out glandular fever as a cause.

The possible role of tuberculous mesenteric adenitis has been discussed already (p. 35). Occasionally children complain of transient attacks of pain with a primary tuberculous infection, and in rare cases tuberculous adenitis may produce pain associated with partial obstruction.

In two cases not in the present series tuberculous mesenteric adenitis with calcification did cause pain, but the underlying condition was readily diagnosable. Both children had recurrent attacks of central abdominal pain, usually associated with vomiting. They were obviously ill and anaemic. Upper abdominal distension and, in one case, visible peristalsis was observed. Plain radiographs of the abdomen showed calcified opacities, and barium meal examination demonstrated gastric and duodenal dilatation. In each case, at operation a mass of tuberculous glands was found in

---

* After the Hospital Series had been completed, an investigation into the incidence of certain *virus infections* was carried out. This was stimulated by a report (Kjellen *et al.*, 1955) that apparently identical strains of virus had been cultured from the mesenteric glands and pharynx of children who had mesenteric lymphadenitis and pharyngitis.

Complement fixation tests were carried out by Dr Paul Mann, Director, Public Health Laboratories, Bath, using lyophilized adenovirus antigen prepared by the Standards Laboratory, Colindale.

Sera were examined from forty-two children within a few days of an attack of recurrent abdominal pain. All were negative.

the root of the mesentery, producing partial intestinal obstruction.

Tuberculous adenitis, like non-infectious involvement of the lymph nodes (e.g. Hodgkin's disease, lymphosarcoma, and neoplasm of any abdominal or pelvic organs with lymph drainage into the mesenteric nodes), must, at most, be a rare cause of recurrent pain.

Masshoff's disease (mesenteric lymphadenitis caused by *Yersinia* pseudotuberculosis or enterocolitis) is an acute illness, characteristically benign and self-limiting (Winblod *et al.*, 1966) though it may be associated with acute ileitis. Culture of the lymph nodes or serum agglutination tests may be positive (1973). A *Brit. med. J.* normal agglutination level was recorded in a random few of my cases in which the serological tests were done.

Ovulation. It was found in the School Series that the onset of attacks of recurrent abdominal pain is common among girls 8 to 10 years old (Fig. 2). It is, however, difficult to correlate this with ovulation, since in this country the average age at which the first menstrual period occurs is 13.5 years (Wilson and Sutherland, 1950) and the first menstrual periods are presumed to be anovulatory (Talbot *et al.*, 1952). On the other hand, the incidence of pains in boys does not show a parallel increase between 8 and 10 years of age. It remains possible that the increased frequency of pains in girls may be associated with increased vascularity and growth of the female pelvic organs in the pre-adolescent years; though if this were so the abrupt cessation of new cases in girls after 10 years would have to be explained, possibly on the grounds that they expect and do not complain of abdominal pains at an age when the menarché is imminent.

Ectopia testis. This possible cause of recurrent abdominal pain has been discussed (p. 34).

Peptic ulcer. In the Hospital Series a peptic (duodenal) ulcer was demonstrated radiologically in only one child. The diagnosis rests on radiological demonstration and the criteria adopted, since the characteristics of the pain and the emotional disturbances in the background may be indistinguishable from those occurring in children without an ulcer (Goldberg, 1957). In many cases, in my experience, the radiological disappearance of an ulcer occurs very quickly, often without any form of treatment and with little or no relation to pain.

It has been affirmed that peptic ulcer is a relatively common condition in childhood (Prouty, 1967). Wood and her colleagues (1955) diagnosed duodenal ulcer in six of ninety-five children with recurrent abdominal pains, and Alexander (1951) in thirty of 254 cases. Barium meal examination is not carried out routinely in my cases, but among those (usually with severe epigastric pain or with a family history of confirmed peptic ulcer) in whom it is done, the proportion is very small, and in a considerable series remains no higher than 2 per cent.

Now that endoscopy is being done increasingly in children (see p. 98) the prevalence of peptic ulcers may be more precisely determined. Nevertheless, in adults it has been shown (Brown *et al.*, 1972) that there is a poor relationship between ulcer healing and symptoms and Hunt (1973) affirms that the presence of an ulcer has little relation to duodenal symptoms.

Aerophagy. Two examples were found in the Hospital Series (p. 36), though in standard text-books this phenomenon is described only in infancy. In two additional cases the child complained of a 'tight feeling' with attacks of pain, relieved by loosening the clothes and, in one instance, by passing flatus; but in these the possibility of air-swallowing could not be confirmed. In all these children there were marked emotional disturbances, with which aerophagy was considered to be associated. If this is so these cases should be allocated to the 'non-organic' group.

Miscellaneous disorders
Spinal disease. In the past most clinicians will have encountered tuberculous disease of the spine presenting with recurrent abdominal pain (see p. 38). It should be readily diagnosable on clinical and radiological evidence. I have seen von Recklinghausen's disease (multiple neurofibromatosis) present similarly. *Discitis* is another rare cause but may occur in childhood.

JONATHAN I., *aged 4, was admitted to hospital with a diagnosis of ? appendicitis. He had suffered from mild central abdominal pain previously but this time it was severe. He woke several times in the night and screamed if he was moved or sat up. The lower spine was held rigid and an X-ray showed narrowing of the L2–L3 intervertebral space with irregularity of the end-plate of L2.*

Allergic disorders. Children with anaphylactoid purpura may suffer for long periods from recurrent abdominal pain. As the sole symptom, however, it would be extraordinary; almost invariably purpuric manifestations occur in the skin at some time, and examination of the stools and urine may reveal frank or occult blood.

In *hereditary angioneurotic oedema* attacks of abdominal pain may occur. No allergic cause has been demonstrated but recent work (Sheldon *et al.*, 1967) indicates that most of the patients lack an alpha-2 globulin or it is functionally inactive.

Children with gastro-intestinal allergy, possibly associated with food sensitivity, may suffer from abdominal pains (Hoefer *et al.*, 1951), and eosinophils can be found in the stools and in the blood. In none of my few cases investigated on these lines were these criteria fulfilled. Nor, in my complete group of cases, was there evidence of an increased tendency to allergic disorders or of food sensitivity. In infants, particularly under 6 months of age, recurrent abdominal pain can be due to *lactose intolerance* but less rarely to a milk protein allergy. It is likely to be associated with chronic diarrhoea and failure to thrive, and the infant responds quickly to a lactose-free soya preparation (Holzel, 1973). In 5 otherwise healthy children abdominal pains are reported to have been reproduced by lactose tolerance tests and abated by a partial reduction of milk and lactose (Bayless and Huang, 1971); in my own patients (p. 10) lactose tolerance tests have not contributed.

I have heard it suggested that the incidence of recurrent abdominal pains is proportional to the amount of milk consumed; but a comparison of the amount of milk consumed among children in the School Series and controls showed little difference. Indeed, the children with pains were as finicky about taking milk as about other foods. The possibility that dietary abnormalities of any sort play a significant part in the pathogenesis of any but the most trivial of abdominal pains has not been confirmed in these studies.

Metabolic disorders. In those of my cases in which pains occurred predominantly on an empty stomach, glucose tolerance tests were done. Following on Cameron's (1946) description it has been recognized that functional hypoglycaemia is liable to occur in nervous, thin children prone to alimentary upsets. The hypoglycaemic attacks tend to occur not only on an empty stomach but with excitement of anxiety (Conn, 1947). For diagnosis a single blood-sugar estimation is fallacious: following a high carbohydrate

diet for 3 days beforehand, it is necessary to demonstrate a fall of
blood sugar to hypoglycaemic levels 3 to 4 hours after glucose has
been given. In the cases in which this test was done the results
were normal. None of the children with pain had diabetes
mellitus, which would be expected to have become evident before
a period of 3 months with pains had elapsed. The spectroscopic
examination of urine for porphyrins was carried out because of the
rare association of recurrent abdominal pain with porphyrinuria,
but in my series the examination was invariably negative.

PRISCILLA E. (*Case of Dr J. J. Kempton, quoted by kind permission.*) *A 13-year-old girl, complaining for a year of recurrent attacks
of abdominal pain with headache, vomiting and pyrexia. Dark
urine had been noticed, but was thought to be due to concentration
occurring with fever; the urine had been reported as normal on routine
examination on two previous hospital admissions. When admitted to
hospital at the onset of a later attack, she was found to have acute
idiopathic porphyrinuria. Since then a further episode has been
associated with numbness and tingling of the feet.*

Hyperbilirubinaemia. Patients with the rare Gilbert's disease
(familial unconjugated hyperbilirubinaemia) may suffer from vague
abdominal pain, nausea and anxiety, *inter alia*. A raised serum
bilirulin level may be found though it fluctuates considerably.

IN SUSAN C., *aged 5, the serum bilirubin rose to 5.9 g at times,
but one could not be sure how much the concern surrounding her
condition contributed to the symptoms of pain and anxiety.*

Idiopathic familial hyperlipaemia (fat induced) occurs usually in
children under 10 years, and is characterized by attacks of abdominal pain and hepatosplenomegaly, which may suggest the diagnosis. Fever and peritoneal irritation may also occur (Frederickson and Lees, 1966).

Lead poisoning. Chronic lead poisoning itself is rare, though
hazards from environmental pollution are being increasingly
recognized (Lansdown *et al.*, 1974). Abdominal colic from this
cause is probably even less common in children than in adults.
The diagnosis may be confirmed or excluded by examination of
blood and urine and bone X-rays.

Chapter 9
Other Causes.
Pathogenesis of Abdominal Pain

Miscellaneous recurrent disorders. Epilepsy. Emotional
disturbances. The pathogenesis of recurrent abdominal pain

The position of abdominal pain in the group of recurrent disorders, and the role of epilepsy and of emotional disorders in pathogenesis, will be discussed in this chapter.

MISCELLANEOUS RECURRENT DISORDERS

The original description of periodic disorders is generally attributed to Samuel Gee (1882) who, succinctly describing nine cases of 'fitful or recurrent vomiting' with abdominal pain and fever in children, remarked: 'These cases seem to be all of the same kind.' He was, however, anticipated by Heberden, whose description of recurrent abdominal pain appeared in *Commentaries on the History and Cure of Diseases* (1802). Heberden wrote: 'Beside the pains which are either constantly felt, or rage at certain times, there are others which are regularly intermittent; such I have known in the bowels, stomach . . .' Such apparently unrelated disturbances as recurrent vomiting, abdominal pain, fever, and headache, were collated and unified by Wyllie and Schlesinger (1933), whose important conception of 'The periodic group of disorders' was expanded and elaborated by Reimann (1951). To Wyllie and Schlesinger's tetrad may be added diurnal limb pains (Naish and Apley, 1951), as suggested by Mac Keith (1955). It would, however, seem to be applying the conception indiscriminately, and thereby destroying its significance, if such diverse conditions as familial periodic paralysis, intermittent hydrarthrosis, periodic neutropenia, haemolytic (auto-immune) anaemia, and the like, were to be included because they are characterized *inter alia* by periodicity.

Recent trends are exemplified, first, by Moore (1945 and 1950), Livingston (1951) and Wallis (1955b), and by Farquhar (1956), who, under the designations of abdominal epilepsy and abdominal migraine, have revived a suggestion of Frederick Still (1912) and emphasize epilepsy in pathogenesis; and, second, by Mac Keith and O'Neill (1951) who have reported valuable studies on the role of emotional disturbances. Franklin (1952), Mac Keith (1955), Kempton (1956) and others have made a welcome contribution by reiterating the necessity for perspective in diagnosis, and by emphasizing the theme of common underlying factors.

Though 'periodic' implies regularity of recurrence, in the Periodic Syndrome there is often considerable irregularity; furthermore, the components of the syndrome may be variable and interchangeable. In paediatric practice such observations are common and are recorded by many of the authors cited in this section. For example, Kempton (1956) notes that bouts of pain recede as the child grows older, and vomiting tends to be replaced by headache in adult life. From the viewpoint of adult medicine, I quote Graham, J. R. (1956) from a discussion on 'Migraine equivalents: travel sickness, cyclic vomiting, attacks of otherwise unexplained abdominal pain, etc.' He points out that these so-called-entities occur with such frequency as substitutes for the migraine attack, or as apparently specific disorders early in the life of patients who subsequently develop migraine, that they may be considered as closely related. Nevertheless, recurrent abdominal pains in childhood do not respond to ergotamine (Graham, J. G., 1969).

From such recorded observations, and from the variations in symptomatology noted in the Hospital Series (Chap. 4) and in the follow-up survey (Table 5), I have come to regard recurrent abdominal pain as one part of a wide spectrum of disorder, in which the Periodic Syndrome is included, varying from one patient to another and chronologically in an affected individual. In different parts of the spectrum, standing out boldly as the primary colours, sharply outlined features may be recognized and named; but between them the manifestations of disorder merge into one another.

With this approach the pseudo-problem reflected in fruitless terminological arguments between 'acidosis', cyclical vomiting, abdominal epilepsy, abdominal migraine and the like, is avoided.*

Underlying disorders
In the search for an underlying pathology among the many children in whom no organic disorder is demonstrable, two factors have received considerable attention in recent years: epilepsy and emotional disorder.

EPILEPSY

A clinical impression that paroxysmal visceral disturbances may be variants, or equivalents, of unsuspected epilepsy has long been current, and has apparently been strengthened by some publications on 'abdominal epilepsy'. Attention is, however, drawn to the fact, sometimes over-looked, that in many reported cases of abdominal epilepsy unmistakable epileptic manifestations also occurred. Thus, in Trousseau's case (1868), the first recorded, sudden attacks of 'pressure in the pit of the stomach soon followed by vomiting' were accompanied by 'momentary impairment of the intellect'. More recently, of Moore's (1945) cases of abdominal epilepsy, all but one had clinical features indicative of overt epilepsy; and, among Millichap's (1955) thirty-three cases of cyclical vomiting (of whom half also complained of abdominal pain), four were mentally retarded and fourteen had a history of fits or loss of consciousness. When conclusions are derived from what is often admittedly selected material their general applicability is difficult to evaluate; I propose to discuss the evidence for and against an association between epilepsy and recurrent abdominal pain from two broader aspects.

---

* The more superficial disadvantages of each term can be briefly stated:
   Acidosis is not a diagnosis and, in the present context, is simply incorrect. The term should be reserved for those rare disorders in which there is an accumulation of acid or depletion of base in the body.
   Cyclical vomiting is too narrow a term, though it has the merit of avoiding aetiological assumptions. An attack may often last for days, instead of for minutes or hours with the typical bout of abdominal pain.
   Abdominal epilepsy implies a serious disorder, often unproven, and the term may itself provoke unfortunate personal, familial and social reactions.
   Abdominal migraine is self-contradictory, for migraine comes from the Latin *hemicrania* meaning '(pain in) the half of the head'.

Pain in children with overt epilepsy

In a proportion of children with overt epilepsy fits are preceded by pain in the abdomen or elsewhere. It would therefore be reasonable to expect that in some instances pain, as a manifestation of an incomplete or abortive epileptic disturbance, would occur alone.* To support this possibility, epileptic subjects should be unduly prone to attacks of pain, unassociated with frank epileptic manifestations.

I have been unable to find any figures to demonstrate the frequency with which pain, unassociated with fits, occurs in epileptic children; inquiries were therefore made among a hundred consecutive children, at least 3 years old, with undoubted epilepsy. The results are summarized in Table 19.

INCIDENCE OF PAIN

Among a hundred children with overt epilepsy, therefore, recurrent pain occurred predominantly in the head in twenty, in the abdomen in fourteen, and in the limbs in three.

I have found no comparable figures for the frequency of headaches in non-epileptic children, though headache is undoubtedly common and is one of the the three most frequent reasons given for repeated absence from school (Bransby, 1951) in this country. [In a large Swedish survey of children from 7 to 15 years old the following figures were reported: 3.9 per cent with migraine, 6.8 per cent with frequent and 48.0 per cent with infrequent non-migrainous headaches, while the remaining 41.4 per cent had no headaches (Bille, 1967)]. The incidence of limb pains is slightly lower and that of abdominal pains is rather higher (p. 23) than among unselected schoolchildren (Naish and Apley, 1951); but it must be borne in mind that recurrent pain among all children attending hospital (as were the group of epileptic children under discussion) is certainly commoner than among unselected schoolchildren.

Moreover, in children suffering from fits, it may be incorrect to assign attacks of pain directly to the epileptic disturbance; they may be associated with emotional disturbances. Thus, Bridge (1949) found that one-third of a large group of epileptic children

---

* Among 8000 children attending an epileptic clinic Livingston (1956) diagnosed abdominal epilepsy in thirty-two (0.4 per cent).

were mildly disturbed emotionally and 9 per cent were severely disturbed.

EFFECTS OF TREATMENT

In the majority of the fourteen epileptic children with recurrent abdominal pain, this symptom ceased or was considerably improved when the fits were controlled by drug therapy. But in two cases attacks of abdominal pain persisted unchanged after the fits ceased; and in one case severe attacks of abdominal pain commenced after the fits had been controlled with drugs.*

Table 19. Pain unassociated with fits in epileptic children*

Predominant clinical type of epilepsy	Number of children	Recurrent pain predominantly in		
		Head	Abdomen	Limbs
Grand mal	61	10	8	2
Petit mal	31	6	5	1
Ungrouped	8	4	1	0
Total	100	20	14	3

* In five of the thirty-seven children affected pain occurred variably in the head, abdomen or limbs, and in one abdominal pain had been replaced by headache. In two cases (not included in the table) abdominal pain, recurring for 2 to 3 years, had ceased when major epileptic attacks developed.

SUBSTITUTION OF PAIN BY FITS

Among the group of a hundred epileptic children there were two in whom recurrent abdominal pain ceased when major epilepsy commenced. Similar observations are frequently recorded in publications of the anecdotal type, and it would be comparatively easy to collect a number of such instances. Against this must be set the large number of children in whom abdominal pain occurs; the development of epilepsy in a small proportion of them would

* A high rate of 'cures' in children with recurrent abdominal pain has been claimed for drugs which have little effect on petit mal. Yet, as Table 19 shows, in a considerable proportion of epileptic children with pain the epileptic disturbance is predominantly of the petit mal type.

be expected. More impressive, therefore, are such unusual cases as the following:

MAUREEN D. *A girl, 6 years old, referred because of major epilepsy. She had complained of attacks of abdominal pain for several months. With the first major fit a similar pain occurred as an aura. No isolated attacks of pain have occurred since, but each fit has been preceded by abdominal pain of the same character as in the previous isolated attacks of pain.*

Nevertheless, such a sequel is rare. In the long-term follow-up series (Chap. 3) it was instructive to note that 9 to 20 years after the onset of abdominal pain not one of thirty patients had developed epilepsy. Similarly, in the series of 30 treated patients (page 61) none had overt epilepsy at follow-up.

A later long-term study by Papatheophilou *et al.* (1972) is in quite close agreement. The authors wrote to 50 patients who had suffered from recurrent abdominal pain 12 to 14 years previously. 14 of these attended for follow-up and all but one had become symptom-free at about 12 years of age. The fourteenth was the only one who now had an abnormal E.E.G. and he had had 2 epileptic fits at the age of 25. It was concluded from these figures and a further study of other 50 children with recurrent abdominal pain (nearly half of whom went to sleep after the attacks) that 'recurrent abdominal pain seems to be an epileptic phenomenon in only a very small proportion of cases' (see also p. 40).

Evidence of epilepsy in children with pain

In the families of schoolchildren with recurrent abdominal pain a history of fits was commoner than among the families of controls (6 per cent compared with 3 per cent, see Table 3). As against this, in the children themselves the incidence of fits was lower than among the controls (2 per cent as compared with 6 per cent, see Table 4). On both counts, however, the figures are small and not statistically significant. The incidence of 'fainting turns', and of 'blank' or 'dizzy' spells, was the same in groups of children with or without recurrent abdominal pain.

It is generally accepted that E.E.G. tracings characteristic of epilepsy are obtained in 70 per cent to 80 per cent of epileptic hildren, as compa red with 10 per cent to 15 per cent of non-epileptic children. When the E.E.G.s of children with recurrent abdominal pain were compared with those of controls (Tables 9 and 9a) it was found that the proportion of epileptiform and other abnormal tracings was not raised in the group of children with pain.

In some respects there is considerable difference of opinion about the significance of E.E.G. findings (see footnote, p. 39). It is clear, however, from the number of 'abnormal' tracings found in the School Control Series, that E.E.G. variations should not be uncritically accepted as indicating a cause for abdominal pain (Apley, Lloyd and Turton, 1956).* 'As our knowledge of the range of normal has increased, the number of records regarded as decisive has been reduced, and we have been left increasingly to make a clinical diagnosis' (*Lancet*, 1955).

Conclusions

In the very small proportion of children presenting with recurrent abdominal pain, who also suffer from unsuspected epilepsy, a carefully taken history usually permits the diagnosis to be made. Evidence from selected material may suggest that epilepsy not uncommonly plays a part in the pathogenesis of isolated attacks of abdominal pain; but, if the data from unselected children with this common symptom are considered, a causal relationship between epilepsy and recurrent abdominal pain can only rarely be shown.

EMOTIONAL DISTURBANCES

Menninger (1947) wrote that the gastro-intestinal tract 'mirrors the emotions better than any other body system' and, following in the foot-steps of Cameron (1933) and Wyllie and Schlesinger (1933) in this country, and Kleinschmidt (1935), Lambert (1941) and others abroad, there has been an increasing trend to seek beyond the exclusively physical for causes of recurrent abdominal pain in children. Kleinschmidt (1935) stated: 'Undoubtedly the majority of cases of abdominal pain without objective finding have

---

* A similar proviso applies to some interesting attempts to correlate E.E.G. variants with emotional disturbances (Hill, 1955). In children with recurrent abdominal pain (School Series) the proportion of such variants was higher than in children without pain (School Control Series), but further research is essential before conclusions can justifiably be drawn from such material.

a nervous origin', a theme which has been well developed more recently by Mac Keith and O'Neill (1951 and1954). Nevertheless, many contrary opinions persist, and Maitland-Jones (1947) has stated that 'the abdominal expression of psychological discomfort is unknown in childhood'.

A major difficulty has clearly been the tendency for individual investigators to examine the problem of recurrent abdominal pain from a single aspect. Guirdham (1942), reiterating Plato's aphorism, wrote: 'We need the whole physician for the whole patient. Medicine must obliterate its physical and psychological sub-divisions.' In the first edition I wrote: surveys of the problem of recurrent abdominal pain in children which attempt this comprehensive outlook are rare (Lambert, 1941; Franklin, 1952; Mac Keith, 1955; Kempton, 1956). Since then it has been generally agreed in several surveys that an organic cause can be found in only a small (though disputed) proportion. Yet reports and follow-up series in which impressions are controlled and results are compared are still needed. My own earlier views on aetiology, like those of other authors, stemmed from a dearth of precise data and were excessively mechanistic. There had previously been no considerable body of evidence to suggest that there is an increased frequency of abdominal pain in children at times when emotional disturbances occur, or that such disturbances precede the onset of attacks of pain. The data from the present studies have filled some of the gaps and compelled me to modify my views. Subsequent evidence from various sources (Sibinga, 1963; Stone and Barbero, 1970) continues to accumulate.

It is, of course, well known that organic disease may be influenced for better or for worse by psychological factors, but in some disorders these factors play the primary role. To justify a diagnosis of emotional or 'stress' disorder certain elementary criteria should be fulfilled. *First*, there should be negative evidence reasonably adequate to eliminate an organic cause. *Second*, there should be positive evidence of emotional disturbance, and the disorder may be related in time with periods of increased stress. *Third*, though this is not always possible, the disorder should respond to measures directed at the relief of emotional tension.

Absence of organic disorder

A causative organic disorder was demonstrated in only a small proportion of investigated cases in the Hospital Series, and a similar proportion has been found in a much larger number of cases seen subsequently. In a series of 243 cases reported by Conway (1951) the proportion was about the same. Nevertheless, some possible criticisms need to be examined before accepting this low order of incidence of organic disease.

An obvious criticism is that the investigation of cases was not sufficiently comprehensive even by current standards. Thus, Conway's cases had been attended by different physicians, who naturally had carried out investigations for specific indications, according to their individual inclinations and not to a standard pattern. In another large series Wood and her colleagues (1955), reporting a higher proportion of organic disorders among ninety-five cases, carried out standardized, comprehensive laboratory investigations on all their cases, but 'psychometric examination and E.E.G. were done in some cases and further examinations, such as retrograde pyelography, gastric analysis and exploratory laparotomy, were done in those cases in which they seemed indicated'. My own series is subject to somewhat similar limitations. But no doctor can reasonably subject a large number of patients to the entire gamut of diagnostic procedures, even for research purposes, though a representative sample may justifiably be investigated with special objectives in view. In the present studies examples are provided by the tests for brucellosis and porphyrinuria.

A further criticism might be that advancing knowledge will reveal new methods for demonstrating infective or other disorders to account for the symptom under discussion. It is, for example, possible that some hitherto unidentified virus infections may cause chronic mesenteric lymphadenitis and so provoke recurring abdominal pains. A limited investigation into this possibility was negative (footnote, p. 78), a result which might have been forecast because no correlation has been shown between seasonal respiratory infections and recurrent abdominal pain (p. 46). For the same reason other, as yet unidentified, respiratory virus infections can hardly play a significant part in the aetiology of this disorder.

The many observations on altered physiological responses and autonomic activity (see also p. 99) in association with anxiety (Lader, 1970) are relevant to this discussion. If such findings are confirmed they are likely not so much to substitute a physical for an emotional cause of symptoms, as to take us a stage further in explaining the mechanisms of symptom production. Other suggestions of biochemical dysfunction, or of autosensitization to metabolites or secretions, for example, which might provide a basis for what we now call 'functional' disorders, may also be postulated. Thus, the superficial, presenting features of the coeliac syndrome or of porphyria may be emotional disturbances with abdominal pain.

Despite these and similar provisos, and the probability that new causes will be discovered to explain exceptional cases, it seems reasonable to concede that in the large majority of cases no primary underlying organic disease exists.

Positive evidence of emotional disturbance

Criteria upon which to base a diagnosis of significant emotional disturbance are not so clearly established as are those of organic dysfunction—though even for the latter they should not be accepted uncritically (see Chap. 5). It was for this reason, among others, that in these studies children with abdominal pain were compared with controls.

The expressions of emotional disturbance are almost unlimited, but it is unusual for a child with recurrent abdominal pain to present more than a few. Nevertheless, it is the combination of several of these which is, in the majority of cases, clear-cut and convincing, and permits a definite diagnosis (p. 44). In theory, positive evidence should be obtainable in all children to whom the diagnosis of recurrent abdominal pain associated with emotional disturbance is applied. In practice, however, it is obvious that the proportion depends in part at least on the degree of skill and experience brought to the task, and the time devoted to it. The proportion of cases in whom positive evidence was found is shown in Table 13; in the psychiatrist's sub-group it was rather higher.

Where positive evidence is lacking, some help in diagnosis may be afforded by indirect evidence (p. 52). Thus, if stress situations and attacks of pain are obviously sequential, and organic disease is not demonstrable, a causal relationship can reasonably be assumed. Presumptive evidence is provided by assessment of the child's personality (since anxiety, over-conscientiousness, and the like, are so commonly associated with emotional disturbance) and from the family background (emotional and 'nervous' disorders, abdominal pain and related complaints, are unduly common in the families of children whose pain is emotionally determined).

Effects of treatment
Under ideal circumstances, bodily symptoms associated with emotional disturbances should invariably respond to treatment directed to the underlying condition. In practice the results are less satisfactory. Nevertheless, results are encouraging in the large majority of cases (see Chap. 7), even without specialized experience, and compare favourably with other methods of treatment.

. . . . . .

From all the evidence it appears justifiable to conclude that in a large proportion of children with recurrent abdominal pain the criteria of a stress disorder are fulfilled. Organic disease is not demonstrable; emotional disturbances are the rule and, like attacks of pain, are often preceded or exaggerated by a stressful situation; and psychotherapy is usually helpful. In individuals predisposed by heredity or upbringing stress is a precipitating or causative factor. Abdominal pain is potentiated by a failure to adapt successfully to difficulties at home or at school.

PATHOGENESIS OF RECURRENT ABDOMINAL PAIN

'Listening to the child talking with his body' is a delightful description of the sensitive doctor trying to understand a child with recurrent abdominal pain. When the pain is associated with emotional disturbance it is pertinent to ask oneself why the individual should complain of this particular bodily symptom. Even if a complete answer is not possible, many of the gaps are being filled both from experimental and clinical sources. The attempt not to leave the canvas blank, to sketch a broad picture, is worthwhile if only to indicate where important details are still lacking and where further investigation should be directed.

A learning process

The pathogenesis of psychogenic disorders lost much of the mystery when it was appreciated that emotional stimuli can set in motion the same patterns of response as those due to physical, chemical or bacterial agents and that ' . . . almost all so-called stress diseases are fundamentally reaction patterns that also occur in healthy individuals' (Groen and Bastiaans, 1955). Since then the experimental work of Neal Miller has cast a new and brilliant light on the subject. By trial and error learning, using preferential conditioning and biofeedback, he and others have induced changes in the autonomic functions and behaviour of animals and of man. I quote Miller on *Cause of Psychosomatic Symptoms* (1969): 'For example, suppose a child is terror-stricken at the thought of going to school in the morning because he is completely unprepared for an important examination. The strong fear elicits a variety of fluctuating autonomic symptoms, such as a queasy stomach at one time and pallor and faintness at another; at this point his mother, who is particularly concerned about cardiovascular symptoms, says, "You are sick and must stay home." The child feels a great relief from fear, and this reward should reinforce the cardiovascular responses producing pallor and faintness. If such experiences are repeated frequently enough, the child, theoretically, should learn to respond with that kind of symptom. Similarly, another child whose mother ignored the vasomotor responses but was particularly concerned by signs of gastric distress would learn the latter type of symptom.' He goes on to say: 'I have emphasized the possible role of learning in producing the observed individual differences in visceral responses to stress, which in extreme cases may result in one type of psychosomatic symptom in one person and a different type in another. Such learning does not, of course, exclude innate individual differences in the susceptibility of different organs. In fact, given social conditions under which any form of illness will be rewarded, the symptoms of the most susceptible organ will be the most likely ones to be learned.'

I wonder if operant conditioning or preferential reinforcement may help to explain why psychosomatic disorders are so common in our present-day Western society? A hundred years ago if the child had a tummy-ache it would be unusual for him even to be seen by a doctor. Nowadays he will be seen and fussed. He used to be dosed with old-fashioned, nasty castor oil; now he is lured with new-fashioned medicine tasting like ice-cream. He will be kept away from school—is not this preferential conditioning to feel pain? He may be kept away yet again to see a specialist. Perhaps all this is not the best treatment if he is suffering from a passing anxiety state, or even a passing green apple?

From his own observations Meskey (1970) comes to similar conclusions: 'There is strong evidence that . . . the experience of pain depends upon an interaction between the maturing organism and its environment' and 'patterns of pain related to particular areas of the body are learned'. The situation may be summed up in this way: 'We have to remember that psychosomatic reactions are like immunological responses in two fundamental respects: the subject is sensitive to something (an emotional stress or a foreign protein) and his reactions are influenced by what has happened to him before' (Apley, 1973).

The family
All sorts of things 'run in the family'. 'The family transmits chromosomes and customs; it shares genes and experiences' (Apley and Mac Keith, 1968). The behaviour of the child with abdominal pains is based both on his genetic make-up and on the atmosphere of the home. Statistics do not give the whole story, but in a considerable proportion of my cases the children come from what I have called 'painful families'—practising doctors will recognize ruefully what this means. These are families with one or both parents suffering from recurrent pains and psychological problems, recurrent illnesses and pseudo-illnesses. With the background of a 'painful family' the child complaining of abdominal pains is most unlikely to grow up symptom-free (Apley and Hale, 1973).

The abdomen
The gut exhibits a formidable repertoire of psychosomatic disturbances. Psychosomatic disorders tend to follow through childhood some chronological pattern (Apley and Mac Keith, 1968), but the gut is always the main target organ. An explanation is that this is because it is the organ of digestion, of feeding and nutrition, and for children with anxious parents these assume an over-riding importance. Parental anxiety about feeding and the child's reaction to that anxiety can be mutually reinforcing;

attention comes to be focused more and more on the alimentary tract. Miller's 'preferential conditioning' is likely to be most effective in a familial (and social) environment that rewards symptoms and one would expect it to fasten on the most susceptible organ.

An 'awareness' of the abdomen may develop, may be reinforced or almost cultivated, in various ways. It can arise as a habit, acquired from some other member of a family in which pain is commonplace or a dramatic abdominal incident has occurred (Chap. 6). Alternatively, it may be precipitated by a transient disorder during which attention, associated with anxiety, was directed to the abdomen. Deutsch (1939) has shown that in early life the incidence of somatic trauma, such as infection or a surgical condition, may determine the 'choice of an organ' and its dysfunction subsequently. As comparable examples I quote from the present studies: an attack of dysentery or infective hepatitis (p. 33); an abdominal operation (p. 33): and, more speculatively, prepubertal changes in girls (p. 79) or ectopia testis (p. 34). Such factors are obviously likely to apply to a lesser extent in children with a healthy family background and no significant emotional pathology.

Mechanisms

Just as neurology is being rationalized by neurophysiology, so psychosomatic medicine is being rationalized by psychophysiology. The emotion most thoroughly studied has been anxiety (Lader, 1970), which occupies a specially important place in the pathogenesis of recurrent abdominal pains. The well recognized bodily disturbances that occur with anxiety, both in normal and abnormal subjects, include abdominal discomfort. Many of the physiological changes that accompany anxiety have been measured. Yet it must not be concluded that pain is no more than one part of a set of measurable changes: pain is an experience in which the whole person is involved.

A psychophysiological basis for psychosomatic disorders can be outlined in simplified terms (and see Figs 3, 4, 5, 6). When a stimulus makes its impact on the individual a stage of arousal is accompanied by changing bodily states. These all return to normal as the healthy individual adjusts. But he may not adjust healthily, for various reasons: the stimulus may have been too intense or too often repeated; anxiety may have exaggerated the reaction;

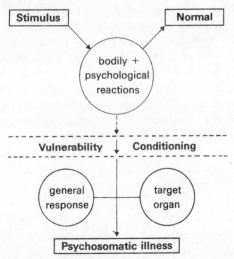

Figure 3. Psychophysiological basis for psychosomatic disorders: composite model (see text).

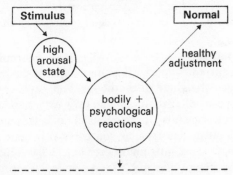

Figure 4. Psychosomatic reations: normal sequence.

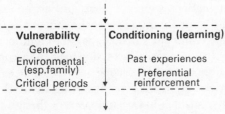

Figure 5. Psychosomatic disorders: vulnerability and conditioning.

through inborn or learned influences, the individual or the target organ may have been particularly vulnerable.

Chronic or recurrent psychosomatic illnesses are likely to be built up on one or both of two major foundations: these are vulnerability and conditioning. In clinical practice such illnesses seem to be characteristically self-perpetuating. There are two explanations: first, a loss of adaptation that is known to be associated with anxiety and, second, an awareness of symptoms (such as pain) which itself acts to increase anxiety.

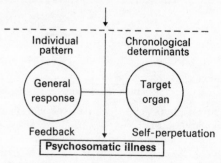

Figure 6. Psychosomatic illness: recurrent or chronic.

Vascular changes

I suspect recurrent abdominal pain to be associated with vasomotor changes elsewhere in the body, though other disturbances (including spasm of involuntary muscle) may also occur. Pallor is a common association of recurrent abdominal pain, suggesting a shift of blood in the vascular compartment. The blood which leaves the skin must go somewhere, and I have long wondered whether it shifts to the gut. Stone and Barbero (1970) have reported on a series of proctoscopic examinations of children who suffer from recurrent abdominal pain (from their report I infer that the examinations were not done during the attacks of pain). They record that in almost all cases the mucosa (up to 15 cm) was pale but with prominent vascular markings and localized areas of hyperaemia. In a few of my cases, in which endoscopy of the lower gut (using a fibre optic colonoscope inserted up to as far as 100 cm) has been carried out, in one actually during an attack of pain, slight and diffuse hyperaemia has been observed. though its significance is not established and it still needs to be checked against controls.

The tone of blood vessels is under the control of the autonomic nervous system and in migraine the mechanism of the attack is an abnormal vascular reaction. Vascular responses to stimulation of the sympathetic nerves may be facilitated by prostaglandins and a direct link between prostaglandins and migraine has been postulated (Colson *et al.*, 1968). This possibility has not yet been investigated in children with abdominal pains. Evidence of a dysfunction of the autonomic system in such children is forthcoming, however, and is based on pupillometry, the measurement of pupillary reactions.

Pupil reactions

The pupil is an obvious though neglected end-organ for the measurement of autonomic function (Rubin *et al.*, 1967). At Bristol my colleagues and I investigated children with recurrrent abdominal pain and as controls we compared them with asthmatics and with unaffected children (Apley, Haslam and Tulloh, 1970; Robinson and Apley). The pupil reactions were measured in the light and the dark, at rest and under stress (a hand placed in cold water). In the patients (a) the pupils tended to be larger, both in the rest condition and under stress, and (b) the changes in pupil size provoked by stress were less (Fig. 7).

I draw attention to an interesting clinical observation. We

Figure 7. Pupil sizes at rest and after stress: (a) in a group of normal children; (b) in children with recurrent abdominal pain (R.A.P.); (c) in normal adults; (d) in parents of R.A.P. children who themselves have symptoms. *Note:* difference in size at rest between (c) and (d) is due to normal decrease in pupil size with age—the age of normal adults was much lower than that of symptomatic parents.

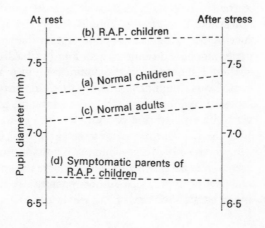

have found a few mothers who had noticed that the child's pupils became larger at the start of an attack of abdominal pain, or at other odd times (see p. 29). One was a 7-year-old boy. When he was sitting in my out-patient clinic his pupils were of normal size. As he went from there to the pupillometry laboratory his pupils were observed to become steadily larger. They were very large indeed by the time he saw the gadgetry (Fig. 8). When he was comforted and reassured they became smaller.

If abnormal pupil reactions indicate autonomic dysfunction one ought to know whether the dysfunction is familial. We have been measuring pupil reactions in the parents of patients with asthma or recurrent abdominal pain. About 20 have been studied so far and many of the parents themselves had symptoms. From our findings (Robinson and Apley) so far autonomic dysfunction may indeed run in the family (Fig. 7).

If autonomic dysfunction is familial, as psychosomatic disorders certainly are, and if it is associated with symptoms, we should not expect too much from medical treatment of the symptoms using present-day methods (see Chap. 7).

Speculations

As a basis for further investigations, my tentative proposal is that conditioning alone may result in recurrent abdominal pain, or other psychosomatic disorders; but that symptoms are more likely to develop, and to be severe and intractable, if there is an underlying autonomic dysfunction.

If recurrent abdominal pain is learned, why cannot it be *un*-learned? If conditioned, why not *de*conditioned? If it can be unlearned the attempt should surely be more promising, and success more likely, in childhood rather than in adult life. Developments in deconditioning, including bio-feedback, may be attempted; but I should expect a significant and practical advance when continuous monitoring using modern instrumentation can be replaced by clinical methods (and intangible awards) which have yet to be evolved (see p. 106).

If the above observations on autonomic dysfunction are confirmed, trials of drugs which can suitably modify the autonomic system should be encouraged, though they could contribute only one part of, but surely cannot replace, a comprehensive approach based on a knowledge of the whole patient in his family setting.

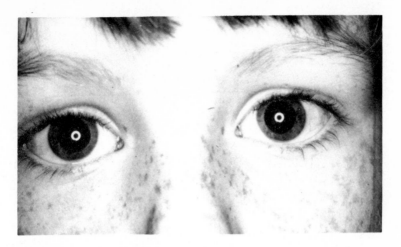

Figure 8. Widely dilated pupils with anxiety in a 7-year-old boy.

Chapter 10
Diagnosis and Management of the Child with Recurrent Abdominal Pain

Grouping of cases. Family background. Emotional disorder in the child. Predisposing causes. Characteristics of pain. Clinical examination. Routine investigations. Indications for additional investigations. Treatment

As a practical approach to the diagnosis and treatment of children with recurrent abdominal pain the following grouping is useful.

I. Organic group
Organic disorders account for less than one case in ten, but prompt diagnosis and appropriate treatment are important. Nearly always they can be quickly confirmed or excluded by a detailed history, thorough examination both *between* and *during* bouts of pain, and a few simple tests. Further investigation is rarely needed, but should be carried out for specific indications. Of these the most usual is a history of abdominal pain which is not central; others are deterioration in the child's general condition or a family history of a relevant disorder.

II. Stress group
In the large majority of children with recurrent abdominal pain the family and personal history, with clinical examination and minimal investigations, provide reasonable *negative* evidence against organic disease together with *positive* evidence for an emotional disorder. With reassurance and informal psychotherapy the pains are usually abolished or relieved.

Even if the possibility of an underlying autonomic dysfunction is confirmed (page 99) this will not detract from the importance of emotional stress, which is indisputably influential.

III. Provisional group

A small proportion of cases, including some with 'false positives' (Chap. 5), cannot immediately be placed in either of the above groups. In these children a trial of informal psychotherapy is well worthwhile, leaving further investigations, physical or psychological, to be considered for those in whom it fails.

HISTORY

The *family history* is important and often extremely revealing. A history of abdominal pain (or severe headache or nervous disorder) in other members of the family is common in emotionally determined cases but uncommon with organic disorders. A history of domestic difficulties or parental illness, including depression, is also contributory.

When the doctor gives parents time to ponder and recollect, important details may come to light. Thus, in my experience, the recollections of a history of migraine may be almost doubled if the appropriate questions are asked a second time, a week or two after the first consultation. A few previously positive histories will then be corrected and cancelled out; but many more will be put forward and confirmed.

Family inter-relationships. It is important to ask specifically what disorder the parents particularly fear in their child; to observe their reactions to the child; and to learn the attitude of the family to the patient and his pains and, indeed, his own attitude to them. Maternal over-anxiety must not be too lightly set aside; but an impression of panic in the mother together with an appearance singularly like satisfaction or 'smiling martyrdom' in the child, often go hand in hand with an emotional disturbance.

In the child, *general evidence* of an abnormal emotional state should be carefully sought, if necessary on repeated occasions. The mother should be interviewed without the child, more than once if need be. Items to note particularly are: a history of early feeding troubles; undue fears, temper tantrums and crying fits; tics, 'picking', fidgetiness, restlessness, and stammering; sleep disorders; over-conscientiousness, and anxiety about school work, or difficulties at school with teachers or with children.

Particular evidence of predisposing causes is more readily obtained than in adults, because the child's world is smaller in time and in content. Details concerning the very first attack are especially necessary. It is worth asking: 'What sort of child is he?', and listening patiently to the reply. Even with a child who seems superficially stable, the mother may come out with: 'he works himself up into a state' or into a pain. But a complete story must not be pressed for or expected at the first consultation. The commonest underlying emotional state is anxiety; the commonest 'trigger' for attacks of pain is school.

The characteristics of the pain, and its associated disturbances, are not often helpful in diagnosis. The child's evidence regarding its site (by pointing to it) is preferable to the mother's, and if the pain is *not* located to the umbilicus or epigastrium an organic cause becomes less unlikely. With an underlying organic, rather than 'functional' disorder, the site of the pain tends to remain constant and pain elsewhere is rare. A serious organic cause can often be excluded simply by the fact that the child is obviously thriving and robust though pain has recurred for years.

A change from the usual site of pain or pattern of the attack should lead to the suspicion of a superimposed disorder, such as acute appendicitis.

CLINICAL EXAMINATION

Frequently repeated physical examinations are unnecessary. Indeed, they may be actively harmful for two reasons: because they focus and magnify the physical aspects, and because they may perpetuate a feeling of uncertainty.

It is rare to discover an undoubted cause for recurrent abdominal pain by clinical examination alone, but when the child is examined the thoroughness of the examination should be made obvious to the parent and the child. While the abdomen is being examined the child's attention should be distracted from it; but, obviously, the examination must not be limited to the abdomen. An additional examination during a bout of pain may be helpful for accurate location of the pain, to observe if bowel distension occurs, and for reassurance than an acute abdominal emergency is not overlooked.

If such conditions as carious teeth, herniae, ectopia testis and lordosis are found they will call for appropriate treatment; but they may well prove to be 'false positives', and the history and examination should be just as complete in their presence as in their absence. A record of the weight may be kept, and a steady weight gain is helpful evidence against a serious organic disorder.

INVESTIGATIONS

Routine

The urine should be examined microscopically in every case, without exception. Abnormal urinary findings, like the presence of leucocytes or red cells, demand further investigation. Plain radiography of the abdomen, preferably during a bout of pain, may reveal stones or abnormal intestinal distension. 'Wantonness in inquiry' must be avoided, and further tests are not advised as a routine measure without additional indications, except (quite legitimately) to help in the reassurance of parents who have some special fear (as of leukaemia, tuberculosis or a known family illness, for example) in their minds.

Additional

Organic disease should, if possible, be excluded promptly for fear that 'the physician becomes a pathogenic agent in perpetuating the illness by his well-meaning but never-ending efforts to find a physical cause' (Weiss, 1947).

The indications for further investigations are, however, rare. Obviously, a child whose general condition is deteriorating needs thorough and speedy investigation. Pallor suggests the necessity for blood examination and stool examination for evidence of bleeding, possibly followed by barium meal studies. Dysuria, frequency, pyuria or haematuria, and loin pain, demand full urogenital investigation. Generalized adenitis or a large spleen call for blood examination and serological tests for abortus fever. When pain is associated with pallor and followed by definite sleepiness, a careful scrutiny of the history is necessary to elicit apparently trivial disturbances of consciousness, and an E.E.G. may be advisable. If pain is associated with abdominal distension, plain radiography during an attack and barium meal studies between attacks are indicated. If the pain is predominantly, or even partially, localized to the right hypochondrium, sub-sternum or loin, the appropriate radiological investigations for gall-bladder disease, peptic ulcer, and especially for renal disorder are advisable.

TREATMENT

Part of the value of a thorough clinical examination lies in the detection of minor disorders, such as carious teeth or lordosis, which may need treatment even though they may not be the cause of the pain for which the doctor was consulted. The fact that the examination was obviously thorough also prepares the ground for a discussion of emotional factors later.

For organic causes of recurrent abdominal pain the treatment should, of course, follow the general precepts of medical and surgical practice; bearing in mind that it is not merely a diseased organ, but a child, a member of a family and of a community, who is being treated.

In all cases, however, whether they fall into the organic, stress or provisional groups, certain principles apply.* Effective treatment starts with the first words spoken at the first consultation. The child and the parents must be made to realize that the doctor is interested not only in the complaint, or in laboratory or X-ray reports, but in the child and his entire background. The more time the doctor spends on the history, the less time he is likely to spend on treatment. It is better to be slow, with a child who remains friendly, rather than quick, with a child who becomes distrustful and uncooperative. When examination and the minimal necessary investigations have been completed their purpose should be fully explained, and a sympathetic explanation of the situation given. But the doctor must be able to listen: if he talks too early he runs the risk of moralizing rather than treating.

Once he has made up his mind the doctor should act confidently and consistently. But it is useless to give reassurance which does not reassure—there should be '*no reassurance without explanation*'. The doctor should not speak his mind too soon. He has to steer a steady course between the Scylla of a cursory examination and a

* The management of recurrent abdominal pain, and other psychosomatic disorders, is discussed more fully in *The Child and his Symptoms* (Apley and Mac Keith, 1968).

hasty pronouncement, which convinces nobody (even himself), and the Charybdis of fitful and frequent investigations which perpetuate doubt and may result in hypochondriasis. It is still easier, alas, for patients, and even doctors, to believe in physical rather than psychological dysfunction.

When organic disease has been reasonably excluded, the aims of therapy are few and simple. Their application is time-consuming but rewarding, and enables the doctor to approach the ideal of treating the patient and not merely a symptom. *First*, it is essential to convince the parents, and to keep convincing them, that the possibilities of organic disease (in particular, of some disease they may secretly fear) have been ruled out. They must also be brought to see that they are not being blamed. *Second*, parents and child should be encouraged to 'blow off steam'. The release of emotional tension may be achieved by patient listening, and by sympathetic discussion of topics about which they feel strongly. Apparently irrelevant details about everyday life, at home and at school, may be of vital importance. *Third*, by friendly guidance they can be shown the way to modify harmful aspects of the child's environment, and so assist in his adaptation. Too often a fancied ailment provides an excuse for comparative failure in lessons, games, or social virtues. Sensible and tactful guidance is needed for an inadequate mother who makes excessive emotional demands on her child, or a father who loads the child with his own ambitions. When advising parents, for example, to loosen the rein, it is helpful to try to discover why they hold the child on a tight rein, and to advise about that. We cannot and should not try to insulate a child from all stresses; but, as far as is feasible, sources of excessive tension should be removed, and the child's and parent's ways of reacting to them should be explained and rationalized. Whether or not the doctor will find it necessary to refer the child (and the family) for specialist advice is a matter, not of principle, but of policy, which he himself must decide.

I am now beginning to try, and ask the parents to try, a rather simple form of 'deconditioning' (page 100) using intangible rewards, like telling a girl patient how much prettier she is and a boy how much tougher he looks, 'now that the pains are going away'. More sophisticated approaches could surely be developed and might prove worthwhile.

Illness is an 'aspect of living, not an isolated episode with a clear beginning or end' and the patient should be treated accordingly. Drugs may occasionally play some part in treatment, but drug therapy may be self-defeating and is at best incomplete. It was Osler who complained of students who came 'asking not wisdom, but drugs to charm with'. Doctors who treat the symptom tend to give a prescription; doctors who treat the patient are more likely to offer guidance.

References

ALEXANDER F.K. (1951) Duodenal ulcer in children. *Radiology*, **56**, 799–812.

APLEY J. (1954) Anal fissure in children. *Practitioner*, **172**, 171–3.

APLEY J. (1958) Common denominators in the recurrent pains of childhood. *Proc. Roy. Soc. Med.*, **51**, 1023–4.

APLEY J. (1973) Which of you by taking thought can add one cubit unto his stature ? Psychosomatic illness in children: a modern synthesis. *Brit. med. J.*, **2**, 756–761.

APLEY J. and HALE B. (1973) Children with recurrent abdominal pain: how do they grow up? *Brit. med. J.*, **3**, 7–9.

APLEY J., HASLAM D.R. and TULLOH C.G. (1970) Pupillary reactions in children with recurrent abdominal pain. *Arch. Dis. Childh.*, **46**, 337–340.

APLEY J., LLOYD J.K. and TURTON C. (1956) Electroencephalography in children with recurrent abdominal pain. *Lancet*, i, 264–5.

APLEY J. and Mac Keith R. (1968) *The Child and his Symptoms: a comprehensive approach*, 2nd edn. Blackwell Scientific Publications, Oxford.

APLEY J. and NAISH N. (1958) Recurrent abdominal pains: a field survey of 1000 school children. *Arch. Dis. Childh.*, **33**, 165–70.

BAYLESS T.M. and HUANG S.S. (1971) Recurrent abdominal pain due to milk intolerance in school-aged children. *Pediatrics Digest*, **9**, 35–42.

BERGLAND G. and RABO E. (1973) A long-term follow-up investigation of patients with hypertrophic pyloric stenosis. *Acta paed. scand.*, **62**, 130–2.

BIGLER J.A. (1929) Anomalies of the urinary tract in children. *Amer. J. Dis. Child.*, **38**, 960–7.

BILLE B. (1967) In *Headaches in Children*, eds. Friedman A.P. and Harms E. Charles C. Thomas, Springfield.

BOYD W. (1947) *Surgical Pathology*, 6th edn. Saunders, Philadelphia.

BRANSBY E. R. (1951) A study of absence from school. *Med. Offr.*, **86**, 223–30 and 237–40.

BRENNEMANN J. (1921) The abdominal pain of throat infections. *Amer. J. Dis. Child.*, **22**, 493–9.

BRIDGE E.M. (1949) *Epilepsy and Convulsive Disorders in Children*. McGraw-Hill, New York.

Brit. med. J. (1955) Chronic appendicitis. Leading article, **1**, 776–7.

Brit. med. J. (1973) Yersinia pseudotuberculosis. **2**, 430.

BROWN P., SALMON P.R., THIEN-HTUT and READ A.E. (1972) Double-blind trial of cerbenoxolone sodium capsules in duodenal ulcer therapy. *Brit. med. J.*, **3**, 661–4.

CARLSON L.A., EKELAND L.G. and ORO L. (1968) Clinical and metabolic effects of different doses of prostaglandin E. in man. *Acta med. scand.*, **183**, 423.

CAMERON H.C. (1933) *The Nervous Child at School.* Oxford Univ. Press, London.

CAMERON H.C. (1946) *The Nervous Child,* 5th edn. Oxford Univ. Press, London.

CONN J.W. (1947) The diagnosis and management of spontaneous hypoglycaemia. *J. Amer. med. Ass.*, **134**, 130–8.

CONWAY D.J. (1951) A study of abdominal pain in childhood. *Great Ormond St. J.* (No. 2), 99–109.

CROFT C.B. and WILKINSON A.R. (1972) Ulceration of the mouth, pharynx and larynx in Crohn's disease of the intestine. *Brit. J. Surg.*, **59**, 249–52.

CUMMINGS J.H., SLADEN G.E., JAMES O.F.W., SARNER M. and MISIEWICZ J.J. (1974) Laxative-induced diarrhoea: a continuing clinical problem. *Brit. med. J.*, **1**, 537–41.

DAVIS D. RUSSELL. (1957) *An Introduction to Psychopathology.* Oxford Univ. Press, London.

DEUTSCH F. (1939) The choice of organ in organ neurosis. *Internat. J. Psychoanalysis*, **20**, 252–62.

DODGE, J.A. (1974). A fresh look at pyloric stenosis. In *Modern Trends in Paediatrics*, ed. Apley J. Butterworth, London.

FARQUHAR H.G. (1956) Abdominal migraine in children. *Brit. med. J.*, **1**, 1082–5.

FLETCHER E. and JACOBS J.H. (1955) Discussion on psychogenic rheumatism. *Proc. Roy. Soc. Med.*, **48**, 66–9.

FITZSIMONS J. (1946) Some observations on non-specific abdominal lymphadenitis. *N.Z. med. J.*, **45**, 248–76.

FRANKLIN A.W. (1952) Periodic disorders of children. *Lancet*, **i**, 1267–70.

FREDRICKSON D.S. and LEES R.S. (1966) Familial hyperlipoproteinaemia. In *The Metabolic Basis of Inherited Disease*, 2nd edn., eds. Stanbery J.B., Wyngaarden J.B. and Fredrickson D.S. McGraw-Hill, New York.

FRIEDMAN R. (1972) Some characteristics of children with psychogenic pain. *Clin. Pediatrics*, **11**, 331–3.

FROMMER E.A. (1967) Treatment of childhood depression with anti-depressant drugs. *Brit. med. J.*, **1**, 729–32.

GARROW D.H. and KANE G.J. (1973) Toxocariasis. *Arch. Dis. Childh.*, **48**, 81–2.

GEE S. (1882) On fitful or recurrent vomiting. *St Bart. Hosp. Rep.*, **18**, 1–6.

GOLDBERG H.M. (1957) Duodenal ulcers in children. *Brit. med. J.*, **1**, 1500–2.

GRACEY M., BURKE V. and ANDERSON C.M. (1969) Treatment of abdominal pain in cystic fibrosis by oral administration of N-acetyl cysteine. *Arch. Dis. Childh.*, **44**, 404–5.

GRAHAM J.R. (1956) *Treatment of Migraine*. Churchill, London.

GRAHAM J.G. (1969) The treatment of migraine. *Prescribers J.*, **9**, 131–7.

GROEN J. (1957) Psychosomatic disturbances as a form of substituted behaviour. *J. Psychosom. Res.*, **2**, 85–96.

GROEN J. and BASTIAANS J. (1955) Studies on ulcerative colitis: personality structure, emotional conflict situations and effects of psychotherapy. *Modern Trends in Psychosomatic Medicine*. Butterworth, London.

GROSS R.E. (1953) *The Surgery of Infancy and Childhood*. Saunders, Philadelphia.

GUIRDHAM A. (1942) *Disease and the Social System*. Allen & Unwin, London.

HASLAM D.R. (1969) Age and the perception of pain. *Psychon. Sci.*, **15**, 86–7.

HEBERDEN W. (1802) *Commentaries on the History and Cure of Disease*. London.

HEINILD S., MALVER E., ROELSGAARD G. and WORNING B. (1959) A psychosomatic approach to recurrent abdominal pain in childhood. *Acta paed.*, **48**, 361–70.

HERRMANN K. and SCHICKENDANZ H. (1968), cited Dodge J.A. Röntgenbefunde am magen bei spatkontrollen pyloromyotomierter kinder. *Z. Kinderchir.*, **6**, 34.

HILL D. (1953) The practical application of research and experiment to the mental health field. Conf. Nat. Assoc. for Ment. Health, London.

HILL D. (1955) Electroencephalography. *Recent Advances in Neurology and Neuropsychiatry*, 6th edn. Churchill, London.

HOEFER P.F.A., COHEN S.M. and GREELEY D.M. (1951) Paroxysmal abdominal pain. *J. Amer. med. Ass.*, **147**, 1–6.

HOLZEL A. (1973) Personal communication.

HUNT T.C. (1972) Digestive disease—the changing scene. *Brit. med. J.*, **4**, 689–94.

HYDE J.S., SWARTS C.L., NICHOLAS E.E., SNEAD C.R. and STRASSER N.F. (1963) Superior mesenteric artery syndrome. *Amer. J. Dis. Child.*, **106**, 25–34.

ILLINGWORTH R.S. (1971) *The Treatment of the Child at Home*. Blackwell Scientific Publications, Oxford.

KEMPTON J.J. (1956) The periodic syndrome. *Brit. med. J.*, **1**, 83–6.

KEYNAN A., HARDOFF D., BERGER A. and WINTER S. (1973) *The Family Physician*, **3**, 1–8.

KJELLEN L., LAGERMALM G., SVEDMYR A. and THORSSON K.G. (1955). Crystalline-like patterns in the nuclei of cells infected with an animal virus. *Nature*, **175**, 505–6.

KLEINSCHMIDT H. (1935) *Diseases of Children*, ed. von Pfaundler M. and Schlossman A., vol. IV. Lippincott, Philadelphia.

LACEY G. (Personal communciation.)

LACEY J.I. (1958) Conf. on research on stress in relation to mental health and mental illness, Oxford.

LADER M. (1970) Psychosomatic and psychophysiological aspects of anxiety. In *Modern Trends in Psychosomatic Medicine* (2). Butterworth, London.

LAMBERT J.P. (1941) Psychiatric observations on children with abdominal pain. *Amer. J. Psychiat.*, **98**, 451–4.

Lancet (1955) Vasomotor headache and epilepsy. Annotation, **ii**, 913–4.

Lancet (1969) The irritable bowel, **ii**, 1112–4.

LANSDOWN R.G., CLAYTON B.E., GRAHAM P.J., SHEPHERD J., DELVES H.T. and TURNER W.C. (1974) Blood levels, behaviour and intelligence: a population study. *Lancet*, **i**, 538–41.

LIVINGSTON S. (1951) Abdominal pain as a manifestation of epilepsy. *J. of Pediatr.*, **38**, 687–95.

LIVINGSTON S. (1953) What is pain? *Sci. Amer.*, **188**, 59–66.

LIVINGSTON S. (1956) *Year Book of Pediatrics*, ed. Gellis S.S., The Year Book Publishers, 1956-1957 Series, 418–20.

MAC KEITH R. (1953) Poussées fébriles à repetition chez les enfants. *Arch. fr. Pédiat.*, **10**, 176.

MAC KEITH R. (1955) The psychosomatic approach in paediatrics. In *Modern Trends in Psychosomatic Medicine*, Butterworth, London.

MAC KEITH R. and O'NEILL D. (1951) Recurrent abdominal pain in children. *Lancet*, **ii**, 278–82.

MAC KEITH R. and O'NEILL D. (1954) The management of recurrent stress disorders in children. *Practitioner*, **172**, 37–48.

MAITLAND-JONES A.G. (1947) *Diseases of Children*, Garrod, Batten and Thursfield, ed. Paterson D. and Moncrieff, A. 4th edn. Arnold, London.

MELZACK R. and SCOTT T.H. (1957) The effects of early experience on the response to pain. *J. comp. Pathol.*, **50**, 155.

MENNINGER, W.C. (1947) Psychosomatic medicine, somatization reactions. *Psychosom. Med.*, **9**, 92–7.

MERSKEY H. (1970) On the development of pain. *Headache*, **10**, 116-23.

MILLER N.E. (1969) Learning of visceral and glandular responses. *Science*, **163**, 434–45.

MILLICHAP J.G., LOMBROSO C.T. and LENNOX W.G. (1955) Cyclic vomiting as a form of epilepsy in children. *Pediatrics*, **15**, 705–14.

MOORE M.T. (1945) Paroxysmal abdominal pain. *J. Amer. med. Ass.*, **129**, 1233–40.

MOORE M.T. (1950) Abdominal epilepsy: a clinical entity. *Amer. J. Med. Sci.*, **220**, 87–90.

NAISH J.M. and APLEY J. (1951) Growing pains: a clinical study. *Arch. Dis. Childh.*, **26**, 134–40.

NASH F.W. (1971) Familial calcific pancreatitis. *Proc. Roy. Soc. Med.*, **64**, 17.

O'NEILL D. (1958) Stress and disease: a review of principles. *Brit. med. J.*, **2**, 285–7.

PAPATHEOPHILOU R., JEAVONS P.M. and Disney M.E. (1972) Recurrent abdominal pain: a clinical and electroencephalographic study. *Devel. Med. Child. Neurol.*, **14**, 31–44.

PENNER D.W. (1949) Acute non-specific mesenteric adenitis. *Manitoba Med. Rev.*, **29**, 275-6.

PRINGLE M.L.K., BUTLER N.R. and DAVIE R. (1966) 11,000 Seven Year Olds (1st Report of National Child Devel. Study). Longmans.

PROUTY M. (1967) Ulcers in childhood. *Pediatrics Digest*, **9**, 35-42.

REIMANN H.A. (1951) Periodic disease. *Medicine*, **30**, 219-45.

REIMANN H.A., MOADIE J., SEMERDJIAN S. and SAHYOUN P.F. (1954) Periodic peritonitis — heredity and pathology. *J. Amer. med. Ass.*, **154**, 1254-9.

ROBINSON J.E. and APLEY J. (to be published).

RUBIN L.S., BARBERO G.J. and SIBINGA M.S. (1967) Pupillary reactivity in children with recurrent abdominal pain. *Psychosom. Med.*, **29**, 111-20.

SCAMMON R.E. (1930) *The Measurement of Man*. Harris J.A., Jackson C.M., Paterson D.G. and Scammon R.E., University of Minnesota.

SHEACH J. (Personal communication.)

SHELDON J.M., LOVELL R.G. and MATHEWS K.P. (1967) *A Manual of Clinical Allergy*. Saunders, Philadelphia.

SHRAND H. and ACKROYD F.W. (1973) Gallstones in children. *Clin. Pediatrics*, **12**, 191-4.

SIBINGA M.S. (1963) Natural history of abdominal pain in childhood. In *Psychosomatic Aspects of Gastro-intestinal Disease in Childhood*. Ross.

SÖDERLAND S. and ZETTERSTRÖM B. (1962) Cholecystitis and cholelithiasis in children. *Arch. Dis. Childh.*, **37**, 174-180.

STILL G. F. (1909) *Common Disorders and Diseases of Childhood*, 1st edn. Frowde, London.

STILL G.F. (1912) Ibid., 2nd ed.

STONE R.J. and BARBERO G.J. (1970) Recurrent abdominal pain in childhood. *Pediatrics*, **45**, 732-8.

STRÖMBECK J.P. (1932) Mesenteric lymphadenitis. *Acta. chir. scand.*, **70**, supp. 20.

STUCKEY E.S. (1950) Recurrent abdominal pain in childhood. *Med. J. Australia*, **2**, 827-32.

TALBOT N.B., SOBEL E.H., McARTHUR J.W. and CRAWFORD J.D. (1952) *Functional Endocrinology*. Harvard Univ. Press, Cambridge, Mass.

TEGNER W. (1955) Discussion on psychogenic rheumatism. *Proc. Roy. Soc. Med.*, **48**, 69-70.

TROUSSEAU A. (1868) Lectures on clinical medicine. New Sydenham Society.

WALLIS H.R.E. (1955a) Tuberculous mesenteric adenitis in children. *Brit. med. J.*, **1**, 128-33.

WALLIS H.R.E. (1955b) Masked epilepsy. *Lancet*, **i**, 70-4.

WARD-McQUAID J.N. (1951) Acute non-specific mesenteric lymphadenitis: incidence and prognosis in children. *Lancet*, **ii**, 524-7.

WEISS E. (1947) Psychogenic rheumatism. *Ann. intern. Med.*, **26**, 890-900.

WILSON D. C. and SUTHERLAND I. (1950) Age at the menarche. *Brit. med. J.*, **1**, 1267 and **2**, 862-6.

WINBLAD S., NILEHN B. and STERNBY N.H. (1966) Yersinia enterocolitica in human enteric infections. *Brit. med. J.*, **2**, 1363–6.

WOLF S.G. (1954) Experimental research. *Recent Developments in Psychosomatic Medicine.* Pitman, London.

WOOD J.L., HARDY L.M. and WHITE H. (1955) Chronic vague abdominal pain in children. *Pediat. clin. N. America* (May 1955), 465–81.

WYLLIE W.G. and SCHLESINGER B. (1933) The periodic group of disorders in childhood. *Brit. J. child. Dis.*, **30**, 1–21.

Index

Abdominal distension 33,37,71,78, 104
Abdominal epilepsy 4,85
Abdominal migraine 4,69,84,85
Abdominal pain, recurrent 3
  age and headache 87
  age and incidence 24
  age at onset 24
  ancillary investigations 5,9–10,31, 104
  appendicectomy and 15,16,17,22, 33,75
  appetite difficulties and 43,95
  associated phenomena 9,28–29
  asthma and 16,17
  basic concepts of 94
  bilious attacks and 16,17
  causes, classification of 68
  characteristics of 24–7,103
  constipation and 16,17,73
  controls 8,10,14,15,19,38,40,41, 42,43,44,47,55
  criteria of 7,11
  definition of 7
  description of 102–104
  diagnosis of 102–104
  diagnostic difficulties 4,5
  diarrhoea associated with 28
  doubtfully causative and incidental anomalies 34
  drug treatment of 54–57,107
  duration of 27
  emotional disturbances and 19, 43,44,89–93,102
  environmental factors 47–52,102
  epilepsy and 9,16,17,34,39,40,69, 85–89,104
  familial incidence of 13–15,95,96
  family and the child 3,13–22,95,96
  family history 9,13–15,102,103
  feeding difficulties and 43,95,102
  follow-up 17–22
  frequency 27
  from miscellaneous disorders 80–2
  from obstruction 69,71,72,73
  from reflex stimulation 69,74–82
  headaches and 16,17,20,21,28
  heredity and family patterning 95,96
  history-taking 5,102–104
  hospital series 7–12
  in adolescents and young adults 18–22
  in children with preceding abdominal disorder 33
  incidence of 23
  investigations 30,31,104
  long-term inquiry 18–20
  material and methods of inquiry 7–12
  mechanisms of 96
  migraine and 19,20,21,22,85
  milk and 44,81
  natural history of 17–18,21
  organic abnormalities associated with 30–40
  organic causes of 31–33,52–53, 67–82,101
  organic group 68,101
  original inquiries 3–63,78,89
  past history of illness 16–17,33
  pathogenesis of 93–100
  periodicity 27,84
  personal history 9,16–17,102
  personality traits and 42,43
  physical examination 3,5,9,96, 103,104
  preceding disorders 33,96
  precipitating factors 45–47,96
  predisposing factors 9,45,94–100, 102
  problems of 3–6
  prognosis of 17–22
  provisional group 102
  raised temperature associated with 28
  referred 71–74
  respiratory infection and 46,74–75, 77–78, 91
  results of treatment 6,32–33,54–63
  School Series 7–12
  severity of 26
  site of 25, 69–70,103
  sleep disorders and 43
  sleepiness after attacks 28,104
  stress group 101
  time of occurrence 26
  tonsillectomy and 16
  treatment of 54–63,105–107

114